ENDING HEAD AND NECK PAIN:

THE TMJ CONNECTION

Randall C. Moles, D.D.S.

MOLES PUBLISHING DIVISION/RACINE WISCONSIN

First Printing	1989
Second Printing	1989
Third Printing	1990
Fourth Printing	1993
Fifth Printing	1994
Sixth Printing	1997

Designed and produced by Jerele Neeld.

Library of Congress Catalog Card Number: 89-090706
ISBN 0-925004-02-2

To Catherine, my office staff,
and my patients. Their care, support, and
encouragement have made this book possible.

ACKNOWLEDGEMENTS

During the writing of this book, I have often paused to reflect on the source of a particular bit of information or on how I had come to embrace a particular concept. This process has reminded me of the contributions so many people have made to my life's journey, one result of which has been this book. I would like to thank all of these people.

The following teachers and mentors have provided the foundation for the ideas herein presented: Ron Roncone, D.D.S.; Ron Roth, D.D.S.; Harold Gelb, D.M.D.; Janet Travell, M.D.; David Simons, M.D.; Eugene Williamson, D.D.S.; Duane Grummons, D.D.S.; Robert Ricketts, D.D.S.; Mariano Rocabado, P.T.; Jeff Bland, Ph.D.; and Lawrence Funt, D.D.S., whose knowledge, wisdom, and encouragement have been invaluable.

The production of this book has also required the help of many talented people: Dawn Tomachek, Janice Connell, and Barb Pope provided word processing; Robert Anderson provided illustrations which gave substance to words; Elizabeth and Jerele Neeld who helped as coaches and editors; and Lee Gruninger for his expertise in designing the cover. A special thanks to writing and marketing consultant Jeffery Lant (of Cambridge, MA) who's contribution was absolutely invaluable.

My office staff continually insisted that I write a book such as this. Now that I have done it, I wish to thank them for their patience and encouragement during the process. Finally, I want to thank my parents, Ben and Sonja, for their encouragement through the years. For without them, the journey could not have begun.

TABLE OF CONTENTS

WARNING—DISCLAIMER

INTRODUCTION

The Blind Men and the Elephant

It was six men of Indostan
To learning much inclined,
Who went to see the elephant
(Though all of them were blind),
That each by observation
Might satisfy his mind.

The First approached the elephant,
And, happening to fall
Against his broad and sturdy side,
At once began to bawl:
"God bless me! but the elephant
Is nothing but a wall!"

The Second, feeling of the tusk,
Cried: "Ho! what have we here
So very round and smooth and sharp?
To me 'tis mightily clear
This wonder of an elephant
Is very like a spear!"

The Third approached the animal,
And, happening to take
The squirming trunk within his hands,
Thus boldly up and spake:
"I see," quoth he, "The elephant
Is very like a snake!"

11

The Fourth reached out his eager hand,
And felt about the knee:
"What most this wondrous beast is like
Is mighty plain," quoth he;
"'Tis clear enough the elephant
Is very like a tree."

The Fifth, who chanced to touch the ear,
Said: "E'en the blindest man
Can tell what this resembles most;
Deny the fact who can,
This marvel of an elephant
Is very like a fan!"

The Sixth no sooner had begun
About the beast to grope,
Than, seizing on the swinging tail
That fell within his scope,
"I see," quoth he, "The elephant
Is very like a rope!"

And so these men of Indostan
Disputed loud and long,
Each in his own opinion
Exceeding stiff and strong,
Though each was partly in the right,
And all were in the wrong!

So, oft in theologic wars
The disputants, I ween,
Rail on in utter ignorance
Of what each other mean,
And prate about an elephant
Not one of them has seen!

John Godfrey Saxe

U nfortunately, today the treatment of head and neck pain is very much like the elephant in this poem: *shrouded in controversy, dogmatism and confusion.* In the ten years I have been actively treating patients with head and neck pain problems, I have seen people who have spent thousands of dollars on tests and unbelievable sums of money on medications. Some of these individuals have even undergone surgical procedures—all in an unsuccessful attempt to rid themselves of head and neck pain. Many of these unfortunate women and men have been labeled neurotic or depressed and placed on heavy doses of mind-altering or anti-inflammatory drugs, to which many have become dependent in the quest of alleviating pain.

It has been my experience as a member of one of the healing professions that the structure of the medical system is one of the reasons why so many problems exist in the treatment of head and neck pain. Quite simply, the tendency toward specialization has created problems in communication and understanding among professionals when a problem arises such as head and neck pain which is influenced by so many different systems of the human body. The patient's "point of entry" into the medical system tends to determine the treatment given. For example, the general physician might prescribe a muscle relaxant; the neurologist, a migraine medication; or the psychologist, a mood-elevating drug or bio-feedback. Some patients respond well to such treatments; however, many do not. This state of affairs is terribly frustrating to physicians, since they are very committed to helping their patients. In an effort to overcome this problem, some doctors have established "headache centers" in many areas of the country. While these centers provide relief for a great many patients, they are often limited by not having "on staff" a dentist trained in the area of jaw dysfunction. Because of this, the centers rely heavily on the use of strong medications to control headaches. For some patients, these medications may only "cover up" the real problem. Meanwhile, the controversy continues over which is the best way to handle the problem of head and neck pain.

In recent years, the term TMJ has become a buzz word for the general public. It stands for TemporoMandibular Joint: a small joint located just in front of the ears to which the lower jaw is attached. Unfortunately, the term TMJ has become a catch-all phrase used for many malfunctions of the chewing structures which may or may not have a relationship to the joint itself. This has created a great deal of confusion, not only in the minds of patients but, also, in the minds of physicians and dentists as well.

The purpose of this book is to help reduce some of the confusion surrounding the causes and cures of most head and neck pain and to establish its relationship, in many instances, to the teeth, jaws and their surrounding muscles. It is my desire that this book will provide the majority of headache sufferers both with hope and with the information that will allow them to become active participants in seeking and accomplishing a cure for their pain.

I have endeavored to simplify a complex subject and, at the same time, to provide as complete a coverage of the many facets of this complex subject as possible. It is my hope that in so doing I have written a book which will be a valuable source of information for those practitioners who at this time are unfamiliar with this new and emerging field of patient care.

CHAPTER 1

Years of Pain Can End

A warm spring sun bathed the gently rolling,tree-covered hills of the valley. Clothed in the skins of animals taken in the previous year's hunt, members of the clan gathered around a fire blazing in a depression of the rock ledge on which they sat. The patient also sat motionless, facing the fire, his eyes glazed and lids drooping from the combination of unrelenting pain and primitive herbs. The doctor placed a bundle of green twigs upon the fire, sending a stream of smoke toward the heavens. Then, he motioned the patient to lie on his side, placing his head on a mound of furs. Taking a sharp, drill-like object from a nearby rock, he placed it just above the ear and began rubbing his hands rapidly back and forth with the instrument between. The patient felt a sharp pain. The hair in the immediate area began to turn a bright red. Soon, the evil spirits would be released and the chronic headache pain, it was hoped, would be gone. Thus, the art and science of headache therapy had its primitive beginnings.

I t is estimated that over half of the people in the world suffer from recurrent headache pain. In the United States alone, between thirty and forty million people suffer from regular headaches. Approximately fifty percent of those patients seeking treatment from physicians have headache pain. The figures are similar for dentistry; between forty and fifty percent of dental patients are also suffering from some type of head and neck pain.

In a study by the Department of Labor, it was found that the greatest cause of absenteeism in American industry was headache pain: over 150 million work days lost annually. Interestingly enough, the next greatest cause of lost time was joint pain: 125 million work days lost. (Later in the book we will explore the connection between headache pain and joint pain.) The cost, not only to the country, but to the consumer as well, is staggering: over $25 billion spent annually in an attempt to alleviate chronic pain. However, an even greater tragedy is the loss to you of life's simple joys and pleasures, due to the intrusion of gnawing, pounding, throbbing headache pain: a dinner cancelled, a birthday party ruined, a vacation punctuated by recurring pain—all speak of your personal loss. There is hope!

MISTAKEN IDENTITY

Medical textbooks traditionally have categorized types of headaches in the following way:

> A. Disease - 2%   D. Muscle Contraction - 70%
> B. Migraine - 10%   E. TM Dysfunction - 8%
> C. Sinus - 10%

These percentages are approximate and will vary slightly from author to author. However, they are fairly representative of the way headache pain has been viewed by the healing professions.

It has been my experience, however, that although this classification is relatively accurate, there is a "missing link." Because of that, many patients suffer needlessly or are treated for years with medications which are unnecessary, due to an incomplete or mistaken diagnosis caused by this "missing link."

A graphic example of this missing link occurs daily in my office. Eight out of ten patients who have come seeking help for chronic head and neck pain, and who have had previous diagnosis of migraine, sinus or tension headache, are actually suffering from a malfunction of the jaws and their supporting structures, commonly referred to as TMJ or more recently as TM dysfunction.

The term TMJ stands for TemporoMandibular joint, the joint between the lower jaw and the base of the skull. The term is somewhat misleading because often the joint itself may not be a causative factor in the head or neck pain problem. Rather, the surrounding muscles may be irritated due to improperly aligned and jaws. For this reason the new term *TM dysfunction* has been recommended by the American Dental Association, because this designation eliminates the word *joint* and is, therefore, less misleading. In this book, I also will use the term TM dysfunction or just TM, because it is more accurately descriptive.

MISTAKENLY MIGRAINE

Every year I see scores of patients who have been diagnosed as having migraine headaches, when, in fact, their problem was related, all or in part, to a malfunction of the jaws or their surrounding structures (TM dysfunction). When these structures become irritated and inflamed, they produce symptoms which mimic many diseases, especially migraine headaches. For instance, a chewing muscle which is irritated can send a signal to the brain requesting blood; and instead of that single muscle's being supplied, the entire side of the head will begin to throb, creating a symptom exactly like a migraine. Additionally, pain from this jaw muscle can appear in the forehead via a mechanism known as *referred pain,* which we will discuss later in the book. The net effect is that you may have been treated for years with migraine medications when, in fact, repositioning of the jaw by the use of a plastic orthotic could very well solve your problem. This is not to say that physicians are not doing their job. On the contrary, they are extremely concerned about the welfare of their patients. However, most physicians were not trained to diagnose this particular dental problem. It is only recently that the relationship of jaw dysfunction to head and neck pain has begun to be unravelled and understood.

THE SNEAKY SINUS

Many members of my profession have found that TM dysfunction problems are the greatest cause of so-called "sinus headaches" for the average individual. Time and time again we see and hear patients complain of having sinus headaches when, in fact, their sinuses are absolutely normal. Surprisingly, the culprit is the jaws, the joints and the surrounding muscles which can refer pain into all the areas occupied by the sinuses. A particularly sneaky culprit in "sinus headaches" is a muscle called the *medial pterygoid* (pronounced me-de-all terry goy'd). This muscle lies deep within the back of the mouth near the borderline of the throat. When it becomes irritated, pain will be felt just below the eye in the area of the sinus. At other times, the *masseter muscle* on the side of the cheek will become irritated, and pain will be felt in the sinus area above the eyes. It is a tragedy that you may be suffering needlessly from these types of headaches when permanent relief is easy to obtain.

An even more unfortunate fact is this: left untreated, *your problems may become worse with time*, leading to degeneration in the jaw joint and even in the structure of the muscles themselves. (See Figure 1.1 showing progression of symptoms over time.)

True sinus problems are most often accompanied by a fever and an elevated white blood cell count. Moreover, heavy fluid build-up in the sinus causes a painful sensation when the head is moved rapidly. If these signs are not present, the probability of a TM dysfunction problem is very high indeed.

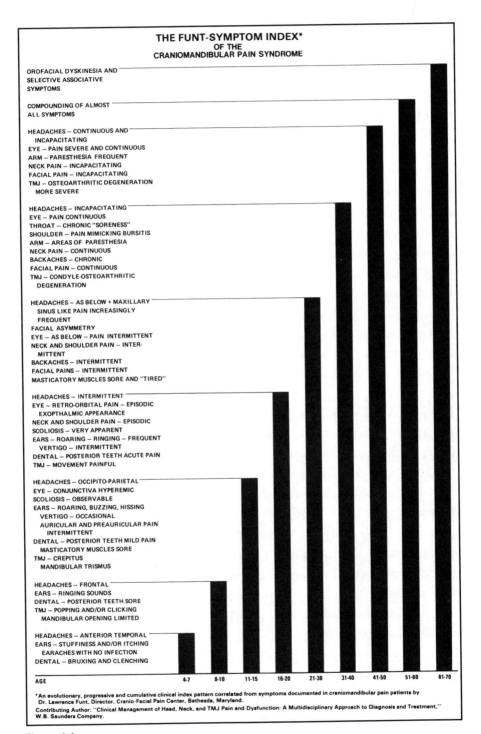

Figure 1.1

STRESS AND TENSION HEADACHES

Many people think that only tension and stress cause headaches. They, contrary to this popular notion, are only part of the story. Often, tension and stress are merely the trigger mechanisms which cause headaches. For instance, when your muscles are already overloaded because they are forced to work harder due to improper structural alignments (poor posture or jaw alignment), stress can add just enough extra muscle tension to trigger a muscle spasm and aching pain. When this occurs, you naturally assume that the whole problem was caused by the stressful situation. This assumption conceals from diagnosis the underlying dental problems which are the main source of the symptoms.

You and untold hundreds, even thousands, of people have been labeled depressive or headache-prone, because the true cause of your problem went undetected. Unfortunately, if a structural problem exists, psychological counselling, tranquilizers or bio-feedback may not prevent significant damage from occurring to that individual's jaw and muscle system later in life.

DO I HAVE TM DYSFUNCTION?

Because of the extremely close relationship of the various structures of the head, neck and face, the malfunction of any one part tends to "spill over" and adversely affect the other components. For this reason, TM dysfunction can exhibit a multitude of symptoms, many of which are seemingly unrelated. Consequently, TM dysfunction has been called the "great imposter." The index (See Figure 1.2) by Doctors Kinney and Funt graphically describes many of the symptoms that have been connected with TM dysfunction.

There is no true "classic" picture of the patient that suffers from TM dysfunction. However, there are a number of symptoms that occur quite frequently:

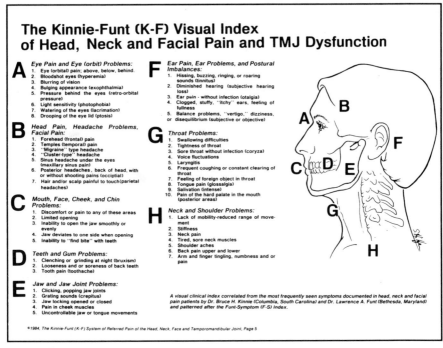

The figure shows:

The Kinnie-Funt (K-F) Visual Index of Head, Neck and Facial Pain and TMJ Dysfunction

A Eye Pain and Eye (orbit) Problems:
1. Eye (orbital) pain; above, below, behind.
2. Bloodshot eyes (hyperemia)
3. Blurring of vision
4. Bulging appearance (exophthalmia)
5. Pressure behind the eyes (retro-orbital pressure)
6. Light sensitivity (photophobia)
7. Watering of the eyes (lacrimation)
8. Drooping of the eye lid (ptosis)

B Head Pain, Headache Problems, Facial Pain:
1. Forehead (frontal) pain
2. Temples (temporal) pain
3. "Migraine" type headache
4. "Cluster-type" headache
5. Sinus headache under the eyes (maxillary sinus pain)
6. Posterior headaches, back of head, with or without shooting pains (occipital)
7. Hair and/or scalp painful to touch (parietal headaches)

C Mouth, Face, Cheek, and Chin Problems:
1. Discomfort or pain to any of these areas
2. Limited opening
3. Inability to open the jaw smoothly or evenly
4. Jaw deviates to one side when opening
5. Inability to "find bite" with teeth

D Teeth and Gum Problems:
1. Clenching or grinding at night (bruxism)
2. Looseness and or soreness of back teeth
3. Tooth pain (toothache)

E Jaw and Jaw Joint Problems:
1. Clicking, popping jaw joints
2. Grating sounds (crepitus)
3. Jaw locking opened or closed
4. Pain in cheek muscles
5. Uncontrollable jaw or tongue movements

F Ear Pain, Ear Problems, and Postural Imbalances:
1. Hissing, buzzing, ringing, or roaring sounds (tinnitus)
2. Diminished hearing (subjective hearing loss)
3. Ear pain - without infection (otalgia)
4. Clogged, stuffy, "itchy" ears, feeling of fullness
5. Balance problems, "vertigo," dizziness, or disequilibrium (subjective or objective)

G Throat Problems:
1. Swallowing difficulties
2. Tightness of throat
3. Sore throat without infection (coryza)
4. Voice fluctuations
5. Laryngitis
6. Frequent coughing or constant clearing of throat
7. Feeling of foreign object in throat
8. Tongue pain (glossalgia)
9. Salivation (intense)
10. Pain of the hard palate in the mouth (posterior areas)

H Neck and Shoulder Problems:
1. Lack of mobility-reduced range of movement
2. Stiffness
3. Neck pain
4. Tired, sore neck muscles
5. Shoulder aches
6. Back pain upper and lower
7. Arm and finger tingling, numbness and or pain

A visual clinical index correlated from the most frequently seen symptoms documented in head, neck and facial pain patients by Dr. Bruce H. Kinnie (Columbia, South Carolina) and Dr. Lawrence A. Funt (Bethesda, Maryland) and patterned after the Funt-Symptom (F-S) Index.

©1984, The Kinnie-Funt (K-F) System of Referred Pain of the Head, Neck, Face and Temporomandibular Joint, Page 5

Figure 1.2

1. Headache pain which occurs in and around the eyes
2. Clicking, popping or grating sounds within the jaw joints
3. Difficulty in opening or moving the jaws
4. Ear pain without infection
5. Hearing changes such as ringing, diminished hearing or a clogged, stuffy feeling
6. Dizziness
7. Neck pain
8. Sinus-type pain under the eyes

If you have one or more of the above symptoms, there is a strong possibility that at least part of your problem may be related to a dysfunction of your jaw structures. Moreover, if your problem has continued despite the efforts of your physician to provide relief, an evaluation by a professional trained in the areas of jaw dysfunction and head and neck pain would certainly be advisable.

HOW BAD CAN IT HURT?

Pain from TM dysfunction can ruin your day; it can ruin your week; it can ruin your month; it can even ruin your whole life. Headache pain has destroyed relationships, caused jobs to be lost, and has even driven people to take their own lives. People will do almost anything to get rid of headache pain.

As far back as the neolithic age, trephining (drilling holes in the head to allow evil spirits to escape) was practiced in hope of curing headache pain. The ancient Egyptians applied a poultice of moist mortar to the head in order to rid the individual of evil spirits. (However, it is most likely that the coolness of the mortar is what provided some relief.) Through the years, various combinations of herbs have been applied externally and have been taken internally. During the Middle Ages, even blood-letting and leeches applied to various parts of the body were used to treat headaches. As civilization moved into the twentieth century, pain relief could be provided through the use of drugs. However, little could be done to provide a permanent cure for headache victims.

Today, we are in the middle of a revolution which can provide relief from head and neck pain to millions of individuals. This has occurred because of a new awareness of the intimate relationship of the jaws and their supporting structures to the overall well-being of the head and neck area. Because fifty percent of all sensory input entering the brain arrives through the fifth cranial nerve—the nerve which controls messages to and from the jaws, their supporting structure, and the eyes and ears—we can begin to understand the tremendous impact that this area has on our well-being. Until recently, the input from the significant portion of this fifth nerve, namely the jaws and their supporting structure, was almost completely ignored in the study of head and neck pain. Today, a new age is dawning; and for many people relief is at hand.

CONCLUSION

In the following chapter, we will look at how your jaw functions, how it malfunctions, and how it can be restored to normal function. We will explore the relationship of jaw problems to aches and pains in your neck, shoulders and even lower back. We will also explore the converse: how problems in your neck can adversely affect the functioning of the jaws.

Symptoms such as ringing ears, difficult swallowing, dizziness and changes in vision can many times be related to TM dysfunction problems. We will explore these relationships. In addition, methods which medical and dental doctors use to relieve head and neck pain, along with these other related symptoms, will be described in detail.

Most importantly, you will be given a method to use for self-examination. This method will help you begin to determine the type of problem you may have. While it is not a substitute for proper medical and dental diagnosis, this self-examination method will give you some idea about the kind of problem you may have and the direction in which you should go to seek help. With the knowledge you will gain from this book, you can seek more confidently the help of those professionals skilled in the area of head pain, neck pain and TM dysfunction.

Chapter 2

TM Dysfunction: What Goes Wrong and Why It Hurts

Jan came to my office at the request of her family. Her jaw made an extremely loud, cracking sound when she was eating. The noise had become so bad that her family had told her if she didn't do something about it, she would have to eat elsewhere! She was also having frequent headaches which she erroneously assumed were caused by her stressful job. Jan was desperate for some relief.

David came to my office complaining of long-standing, frequent headaches and a constant dull pain in the area of his right temple. He said that while he was in college his jaw started to click and that, finally, one day shortly before graduation, it had locked shut and become extremely painful. At that time, his physician had given him muscle relaxants and painkillers. With time, the pain decreased and he had been able to open his jaw, although not quite as far as before.

David also reported noticing that not long after his jaw locked he began to hear in his right ear when chewing soft grinding sounds, very much like the crumpling of paper. Over the years, he continued to have pain, seeing a neurologist for headaches (who appropriately recommended that he have a CAT scan to check for a tumor or blood vessel abnormality), as well as visiting an ear, nose, and throat specialist who was unable to find the cause of his discomfort. Recently, the pain had increased, becoming almost unbearable. David, too, desperately needed relief.

I n this chapter we'll discuss how the joint works, how it breaks down and how that dysfunction can produce pain over your entire head and neck.

If like Jan and Dave you have joints that "click, grate or pop" along with a dull ache or a pain so sharp it feels like a stab wound, you have TM dysfunction. Your TMJ or temporomandibular joint is malfunctioning, creating noise; and when this occurs, the pain comes from muscles trying to protect the joints and the joints themselves as they begin to degenerate.

THE JOINT

Let's begin by discussing the temporomandibular joint itself. The temporomandibular joint is located just in front of the ear. (See Figure 2.1). The joint can be located by placing your finger directly in front of your ear and then moving your jaw from side to side. You can literally feel the lower jaw moving in and out of the joint socket. The upper portion of this joint is formed by a small cup-shaped depression in the temple bone of the skull. The lower, movable part is formed by the end of the lower jaw (mandible). This end is termed the *condyle*. Separating the temporal bone from the condyle is a small, round pad of fibrous material called a *disc*. It is approximately the size of a lifesaver and has a similar shape, but without the hole in the middle. The disc is thicker around the edges and thinner in the center. This *biconcave* shape helps the disc stay in place. Therefore, when this shape is lost the disc can become dislocated much more easily, with painful results.

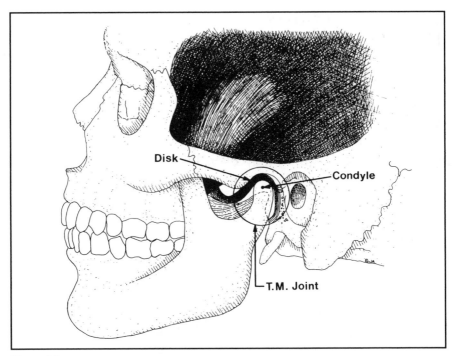

Figure 2.1

THE CAPSULE

Surrounding the entire joint is a sac called a *capsule*. This sac helps stabilize the joint's parts and also acts as a container which holds fluid in the joint space. This fluid is called *synovial fluid*, which is an extremely slippery material that lubricates and also nourishes the joint components. It is 100 times more slippery than the best ball bearing and ten times more slippery than a hockey puck on ice. This being the case, the joint should last forever. Unfortunately, the joint can be damaged easily by accidental injury or constant overload from a bad bite.

There is also a heavy fibrous attachment between the temple bone and the mandible. This attachment is called the *lateral ligament*. The disc attaches to this ligament and forms a very strong bond, thus holding these parts together. When the joint is injured, it is often the lateral ligament which is stretched and torn, allowing the disc or the lower jaw to move out of place.

HOW THE JOINT MOVES

No other joint within the human body is quite as complicated as the temporomandibular joint. This is true because the temporomandibular joint is actually part of a system of joints, all relying on one another and all with the potential for disruption. For example, we cannot isolate the motion of the left joint without taking the right joint into consideration, and vice versa. Moreover, there are thirty-two other contacts (they may even be termed joints) called the teeth, which also affect the movement of the jaw joints. For the sake of simplicity, we will discuss first the normal opening and closing movement of the jaw. (See Figure 2.2)

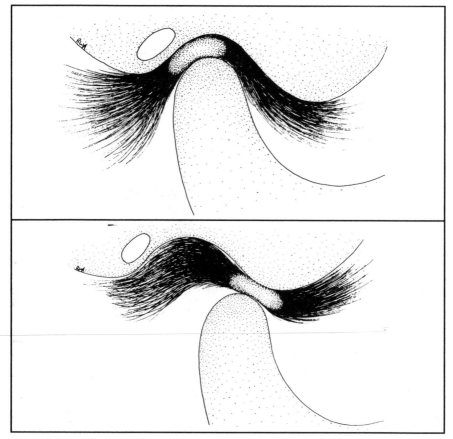

Figure 2.2

When we open our mouth, the condyle (lower jaw) rotates and, at the same time, moves down the forward slope of the little cup on the base of the skull. Simultaneously, the disc moves forward in order to stay between the two bones, thus providing a cushion which keeps the two bones from rubbing upon one another. As the jaw closes, the condyle moves back up into the socket and the disc follows, being guided there by its shape which tends to hold it in place and, also, by the surrounding ligament structure.

Occasionally, as the jaw is opening, the disc may move too far

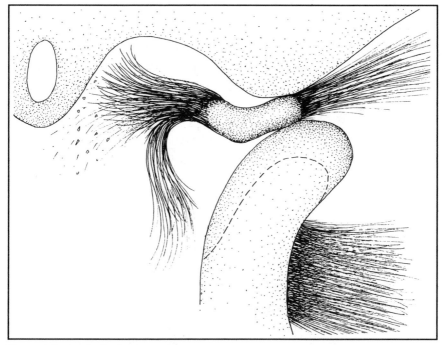

Figure 2.3: Jaw locked open

forward and get caught over the forward lip of the socket. When this occurs, individuals have difficulty closing their mouths. This is called an *open lock*. (See Figure 2.3) If we look at the shape of the jaw bones, it is possible to figure out a method for helping such unfortunate individuals. By giving the lower jaw a slightly down-ward and backward push, we can move the condyle back underneath the lower lip of the socket and into place. (Note to professionals carrying out this maneuver: Be extremely careful not to place your fingers between the individual's teeth since there is a strong reflex action that can occur when the jaw snaps back into socket. The teeth may close very forcibly. If your fingers are in the way—ouch!)

In addition to opening and closing, the jaw also has the ability to move from side to side. When the jaw moves to the left, the condyle on the right side moves downward and forward. The condyle on the left side primarily rotates and moves just slightly to the left. The magnitude of all of these movements is determined by the shape of the joints and also the condition of the lateral ligaments. If the lateral ligaments have been stretched through injury or misuse, the jaw will have a greater range of motion and, unfortunately, will also tend to dislocate more easily.

NOISY JOINTS

When we speak of noisy joints, we often are referring to the corner tavern. However, in this instance, I am referring to jaw joints which make clicking, popping or grinding noises. This is absolutely a sure sign of problems, since a healthy joint makes no noise. Whenever a joint makes sounds, it means that there is friction within the joint. This does not necessarily mean that treatment should be undertaken; however, it does mean that you would be well-advised to have a professional knowledgeable in the area of jaw dysfunction and jaw problems evaluate the noisy joint.

Jaw sounds can vary from a soft pop or clicking sound to a loud pop (recall the opening story about Jan), or they can come in the form of rustling sounds, very much like the crumpling of newspaper (recall the opening story about David). The sounds will sometimes even mimic the sound of sandpaper rubbing upon itself. Each one of these sound patterns comes from one or more specific mechanical problems within the joint. The study of joint sounds has progressed to such a degree that some clinicians are attempting to determine exactly what is going on within the joint by using sophisticated sound-sensing equipment. Although this is in the experimental stage at this time, the use of computers and elaborate sound printing techniques may someday make sound analysis extremely useful in telling us what degree of damage exists within a noisy joint.

The most common noise produced by TM dysfunction is a popping sound of various intensity. If we look at the joint in Figure 2.2, we can see that when the jaw opens and the disc remains in its proper position, no popping sound will occur. However, in Figure 2.4, notice that, because of damaged ligaments, the disc has slipped out of position. Therefore, as the jaw opens, a click occurs as the lower jaw snaps back into position underneath the disc. Then, as opening continues, the disc remains in its proper position until full opening. However, shortly before full closure, the condyle slips back off of the disc creating a soft closing pop. When patients open their mouths and the click is about to occur, they will often feel resistance, a sensation the patients describe as a "catching of the jaw."

Clicking sounds which occur as the jaw is just beginning to open are usually less a problem and easier to treat than those clicks that occur at almost maximum opening. The reason for this is that the disc has not yet slipped very far out of position; therefore, we can assume that the ligaments holding the disc in position have not been stretched too severely. Thus, it may be easy to get the condyle back onto the disc—technically referred to as recapturing the disc.

However, when the click occurs at a much wider opening, one can assume that the ligaments supporting the disc have stretched significantly, making it less likely that proper treatment will be able to shrink them back enough to hold once again the disc in a normal position. This does not necessarily mean that surgery is needed. Many patients can be kept quite comfortable while functioning without the disc in place. However, surgery is one alternative for repositioning the disc if conservative measures do not give suffi-

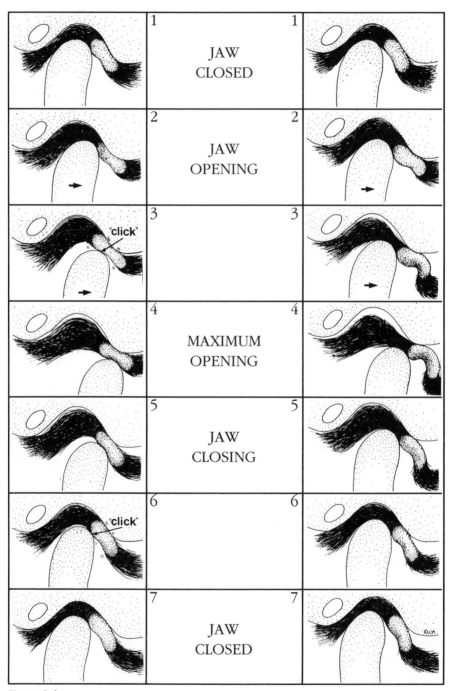

Figure 2.4

cient relief. (We will discuss the various procedures that can be used to treat joint problems in a later chapter.

Although some clicks remain the same for years, more frequently clicks occur later and later in the opening motion of the jaw. This indicates that the ligaments are continuing to stretch, allowing the disc to slip farther and farther out of position. Eventually, the disc will slip completely out of place and the patient will develop what is called a *closed lock*: a jaw which is locked shut. Often when the disc slips out of place the jaw will lock closed simultaneously. Patients report, for instance, that they suddenly woke up in the morning and could not open their mouth, or that they heard a "loud pop" and then their mouth would not open. When this happens, patients such as David often experience a great deal of pain and limited jaw movement, ranging between one-quarter and one-half inch.

Figure 2.4 shows how the jaw and the disc move in a closed lock. Note that the disc never is positioned between the bones during the opening and closing cycle. If nothing is done to correct the slipped disc immediately, then within a few weeks the disc will begin to degenerate and lose its form. During this degenerative time, affected individuals will gradually be able to move their jaw open farther and farther. However, there will no longer be a disc providing protection between the two bones. Once the disc has slipped out of place, the stage is set for continued pain and significant arthritic degeneration of the joint. (We will discuss the possibilities of preventing or reversing arthritis in Chapter 5.) Again, this may not require surgical intervention.

GRINDING JOINTS

Often a patient like David says: "My jaw, which clicked a little bit at first and then with increasing frequency, finally locked one day. With time, the jaw opened wider; however, a dull pain is often present, accentuated by frequent headaches."

This is a very common progression of events which occurs as the disc slips farther and farther out of position, until it finally slips out of place and the patient begins functioning without the protective disc. As a result, the joint gradually becomes arthritic due to the constant rubbing of bone on bone. As the joint becomes increasingly arthritic, there usually is a constant series of painful episodes, depending upon the amount of work the jaw must perform. (Very often, the jaw will be much more uncomfortable after meals.) When the joint has reached this stage of destruction, it is not unusual for patients to compare the sound, as David did, to the rustling of newspaper. That is the sound of bone upon bone and scar tissue rubbing together. In some instances, surgery is needed in order to reconstruct or replace the damaged joint. However, in many instances, patients can be maintained relatively pain-free without surgery or the continuous use of drugs. Later in the book, I will discuss how this can be accomplished.

HOW DO JOINTS GET DAMAGED?

By knowing how the jaw joints originally become damaged, dentists usually can prevent further damage to injured individuals. Dentists also can devise a way to prevent such damage from occurring in others. Currently, research shows that there are two ways in which the joints can be injured: (1) accidental trauma and (2) continual micro-trauma.

Accidental trauma can occur in many different ways. A blow to the jaw in a fall or other accidents can stretch and tear the ligaments surrounding the joint, allowing the disc to begin to slip. An extremely common accidental injury is the whiplash event. Whiplash, which causes violent movement of the head—pushed backward and then forward—can create significant tearing of the ligaments and bleeding within the joint. This occurs because the only point of attachment between the lower jaw and the head occurs at the joint. In addition, during a whiplash event both bony structures accelerate and decelerate at different rates. This often causes wrenching and tearing of the joint structure. If you have had a recent whiplash, please note that the full effect of these injuries may not be felt until months later.

The term "micro-trauma" describes constant, low-level destructive forces which are applied to the joint. One of the most significant causes that has been identified, so far, is the structure of the head and face. Very simply, when your teeth and/or the jaws do not properly align, undesirable twisting, torquing and pulling forces will be applied to the joints every time the teeth come into contact. Because this occurs during the chewing of food and often during swallowing, it is possible for this destructive force to be applied to your joints hundreds and even thousands of times a day. The long-term effect of this twisting, torquing and pulling is a gradual stretching of the ligaments supporting the joint and holding the disc in place. Consequently, clicking and eventual locking of the joint will occur, often with considerable pain!

At the present time, a great deal of treatment is directed toward eliminating or reducing any improper alignments so that further damage is not done. Therefore, it is extremely important, with regard to preventing this type of damage, that children be evaluated at an early age in order to correct crooked teeth or improperly aligned jaw structures. Childhood is the time when the problem most often begins. (A description of how these destructive forces are generated is covered in more detail in Chapter 5 under the section entitled: Facial Structure and Arthritis.)

HEADACHES WAITING TO HAPPEN
From our earlier discussion of headache classifications, you will remember that seventy percent of all headaches are commonly ascribed to muscle tension. These headaches are called muscle contraction headaches, because it is assumed that stress acts on the muscles and causes them to contract, creating the headache pain.

Of course, stress is definitely related to headaches. However, blaming stress ends up much like mowing weeds with the lawn mower; the problem keeps coming back! Obviously, it is necessary to root out the weeds to correct the problem. The same is true of the so called "stress headache," the root being the overloaded muscles which go into spasm with the slightest stress. Therefore, we will explore one of the root problems which can cause the constant, gnawing pain of headaches: muscles that are related to the chewing apparatus, the head, the neck and the spine.

In order to produce chewing motions and the sophisticated movements necessary for speech, a number of muscles must act in coordination. The *masseter muscle* is one such muscle. There are two of theses muscles located on either side of the jaw, running from the cheek bone down to the lower border of the lower jaw. (See Figure 2.5) The masseter is a powerful muscle which closes the jaw. It is only meant to be active when the jaw makes its final closure in a vertical direction. Contraction of this muscle when the jaw is moving sideways can create some truly painful problems. This

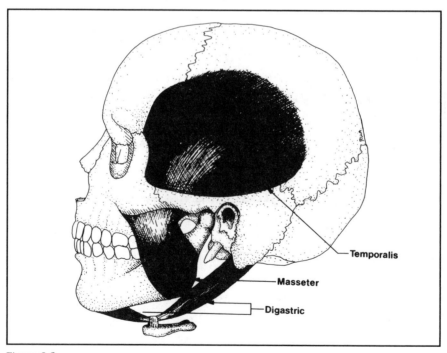

Figure 2.5

improper contraction often occurs when the teeth are out of position and, therefore, do not fit properly.

When a tooth is out of position and bumps during the chewing cycle, the magnificent protective mechanism of our body immediately sends a signal to the brain that says "help me." The brain then sends a signal to the muscles to avoid that particular spot. When a number of teeth are out of position, the brain must order the muscles to execute a sophisticated number of movements just to get the teeth to fit together. As you can imagine, this can set up a situation of chronic muscle fatigue.

In Figure 2.6, line D, we can see the muscle electro-activity as recorded by sensing instruments when the patient has a well-fitting bite. In Figure 2.6, line A, we see a different electrical pattern when the teeth do not fit together properly. This improper fit strains the facial muscles, and before long the muscles will become chronically irritated. Therefore, this person's facial muscles can never fully

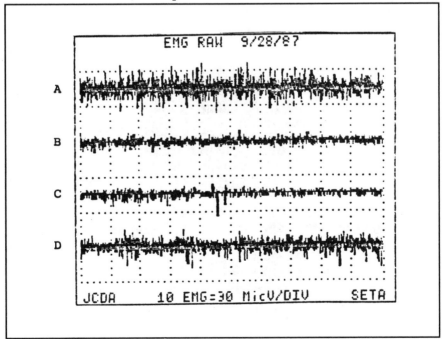

Figure 2.6: Electrical pattern of muscles (Courtesy of Dr. Ira Shapira)

relax. Moreover, even if the person stopped chewing and talking, the muscles would be so tense from the improper bite that they still would never completely relax. This creates a situation where the patient becomes a "headache waiting to happen."

When a patient's muscles are already overloaded, any extra tension within the muscle structure can set off a painful muscle spasm similar to a "charley horse." Of course, as soon as one muscle tightens up, other muscles come to the rescue. If these other muscles, in turn, also are overloaded, they will go into spasm as well. This domino effect can produce a truly horrendous headache!

Another important set of muscles is the *temporalis muscles*. (Figure 2.5) These muscles rest on either side of the head and attach to the side of the skull and to a small projection on the lower jaw called the *coronoid process*. These muscles are responsible for closing and protruding the jaw. It is interesting to note that these muscles often become painful when teeth bump but also can become chronically inflamed in a person whose upper jaw protrudes to a great extent beyond the lower jaw. In that circumstance, the person must bring his or her jaw forward whenever he or she is pronouncing certain words. Unfortunately, this muscle was not designed for that extreme amount of work. (If your upper teeth stick out, watch yourself talk in front of a mirror and you will see that your lower jaw must move forward to make certain sounds.) Correction of this can help headaches and relax the face in general.

In the back of the mouth, behind the upper and lower molars, attaching the skull to the lower jaw, is a group of two muscles called the *pterygoid muscles*. (See Figure 2.7) These muscles are responsible for closure, protrusion and side-to-side movements of the jaw. When they become inflamed and irritated, it is not uncommon for these muscles to refer pain to the area behind the eyes. Because of this, individuals often seek the help of an eye specialist who finds no problem with the eyes. Then people usually begin seeking out many other specialists, neurologists for instance, in order to find the

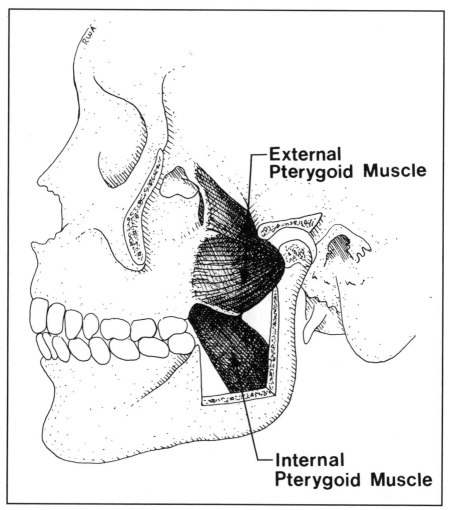

Figure 2.7

cause of the elusive pain. Such pain is often described by patients as a deep stabbing pain. Unfortunately, because of its location, this muscle is occasionally overlooked, even when treatment is given for TM dysfunction problems. However, when properly handled, relaxation of these muscles can give individuals immediate relief.

Below the jaw, attaching the lower jaw to the hyoid bone of the throat, are the *digastric muscles*. (See Figure 2.5) These muscles open the jaw and also greatly help in the production of speech.

Although these muscles are not as often involved in painful TM problems, when they do become tight speech can often be affected.

NECK AND BACK PROBLEMS

There is an old song that goes something like this: The hip bone's connected to the thigh bone; the thigh bone's connected to the leg bone; and so on. The point that the lyricist was attempting to make is that all the parts of our bodies are related. The same holds true in relation to head and neck pain. If the muscles in the front of the head are tightened, there has to be necessary compensating changes in the muscles supporting the head from the back. If this were not true, any tightness in the muscles in front of the neck would cause the head to tip forward uncontrollably. (See Figure 2.8 showing the many interrelated muscles of the neck.) Conversely, when the muscles in the back of the neck are tightened due to injury or posture problems, the muscles in the front of the neck and the related chewing muscles will to tighten in order to keep our head from tipping uncontrollably backward. As you might imagine, this can have an adverse effect on the bite and on the temporomandibular joint.

It is not uncommon for patients suffering from painful spasms of the chewing muscles to also have several neck muscles which are tender to the touch. Studies utilizing spinal x-rays show that when the painful chewing muscles are corrected, undesirable curvatures in the spine sometimes literally will straighten out because of the relaxation in the spinal muscle structure.

The effects of jaw position and neck position on each other can be easily demonstrated. Slowly begin to tap your teeth together while tipping your head forward. You will notice that as your head moves different teeth are touching. Again, tap your teeth together and move your head back as far as possible. Again, notice which teeth touch. Try this from side to side. The intimate relationship of head position and neck muscles to the contact of the teeth will be evident to you. Conversely, when standing straight, if you project

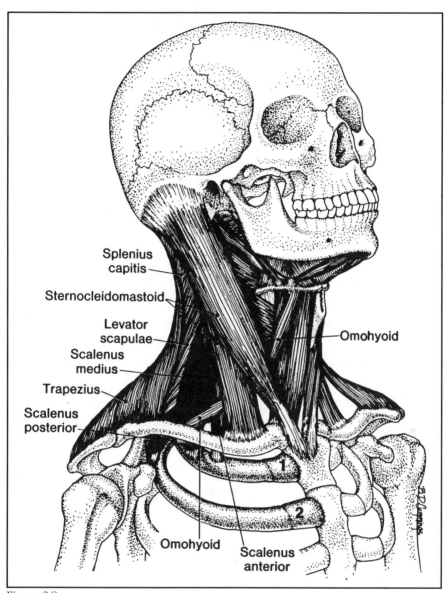

Figure 2.8

your lower jaw as far forward as possible, you will notice that it becomes more comfortable to move your head back slightly. This shows the relationship between the posture of the lower jaw and the position of the head. Because of this relationship, correcting TM dysfunction problems can, and often does, give significant relief from neck pain.

CONCLUSION

In this chapter, we discussed the anatomy of your jaw joint and how its parts fit together when properly functioning. We also discussed the amazing complexity of your chewing system and how it can malfunction causing severe, debilitating headaches. In the coming chapters, we will discuss further how the various factors involved in this complex system come together to create those nagging headaches. We will discuss how your headaches may have been incorrectly diagnosed due to a lack of appreciation for the mechanical functioning of the chewing apparatus. We will also discuss how these problems are of an evolving nature, beginning at a very early age with very mild symptoms and increasing as time goes on. The treatment for these problems should begin at an early age and we will discuss how you can keep your children from developing headaches that rob them of joy and happiness. No matter how old you are, and at all stages of severity, often significant relief can be provided for you. We will discuss the methods by which this can be accomplished in later chapters.

CHAPTER 3

Getting Help: Examination and Diagnosis

When Mary entered my office, she was very skeptical about visiting another dentist for her headache problems. She was even more skeptical of seeing an orthodontist she felt would be concerned only with straightening teeth. Mary had already undergone a number of months of "splint therapy" for headaches which had been diagnosed as a TM dysfunction problem.

Mary had come to my office on the recommendation of a friend because she had not had much success in her previous treatment. Mary described her pain: it was located right over the area of the left temporomandibular joint and also over her left temple. There was almost always a dull pain in those areas with occasional sharp attacks which lasted for hours and virtually forced her to cease working and find a quiet, dark room where she could lie down to get some relief. Mary reported that these headaches had occurred occasionally over the past few years. However, in the past six months, they had become frequent enough for her to seek help.

After examining her, gathering the diagnostic information from her dentist and obtaining some new information in the form of x-rays and models, I saw that only part of Mary's problem had to do with the functioning of her jaws. She was also the victim of referred pain; and, although her dentist had been very astute in diagnosing her jaw joint problem, he unfortunately had not extended his diagnostic evaluations sufficiently to pick up the problems which were occurring in her neck. Within a few months, Mary and I, working together, were able totally to eliminate these recurring headaches.

The one thing that I remember most about Pat was the day she first came to my office, and I sat down to hear her story. In particular, I remember how the first part of our examination took about as long as any examination I have ever conducted, because Pat had been all over the country seeing scores of different physicians trying to obtain help for her chronic headaches. She had undergone dozens of medical diagnostic tests and had visited every specialist she knew of who had even the most remote possibility of being knowledgeable about her headache pain. Almost twelve years later, she still had constant headache pain which "ached and ached and ached and wouldn't go away."

Pat looked at me and said, "I have spent over $15,000 of my own and the insurance company's money without relief. Why haven't they been able to find out what my problem is?" Fortunately, we were able to provide significant relief for Pat. Her headaches were reduced from constant to occasional because we were been able to locate the arthritis within her temporomandibular joints.

Y ou may share this common problem with Pat and Mary: something was missing from their diagnostic examinations which would have revealed the true nature of their problems. In Mary's case, the dentist had not taken into account the possibility of referred pain from her neck muscles. In Pat's case, the physicians who treated her had not taken into account the possibility of localized temporomandibular joint arthritis. These things can easily happen because headache pain problems can have many causative factors which are interrelated and overlapped, thus making diagnosis confusing. Added to this, is the fact that TM dysfunction is relatively new as a causative factor in headache pain. It is easy, therefore, for a diagnosis to be incorrect or incomplete.

Unfortunately, there are many practitioners who have not been trained in the relationships between jaw function and the production of muscle spasm and pain. However, this is rapidly changing; and if you have suffered for years with chronic headaches, a re-examination and diagnosis is certainly in order.

I often tell patients that diagnosing these problems is very much like peeling an onion: when you take one layer off (handle one problem) you often find another layer below (another causative factor). Only after all the causative factors have been addressed and remedied as much as possible can you achieve long-lasting relief. However, when only one part of the problem is treated, symptoms tend to come back with time. Therefore, a complete and thorough history, examination and diagnosis are imperative if your treatment is to be successful.

PATIENT HISTORY INTERVIEW

The word examination can tend to strike fear in the hearts of many of us, bringing back memories of examinations in school in order to achieve a good grade or examinations by the physician when we were younger. However, the examination that I am speaking of takes a somewhat different form, in that the great majority of the time is spent interviewing the patient and discussing the history and the nature of his or her problem. This history gathering is extremely important for a number of reasons.

For instance, it is very important for the doctor to understand exactly what your problem is, when it started, what treatment you have obtained for the problem, and whether that treatment has had any success whatsoever. For example, any symptoms which have occurred within just a few weeks are more cause for concern, since a higher percentage of them may be related to organic problems such as an aneurysm (ruptured blood vessel) or a tumor. On the positive side, if recent headaches can be shown to be related to jaw dysfunctions, then the treatment often can progress very rapidly, due to the short history of the disease. The patient history examination gives the doctor this information immediately.

On the other hand, headache pain which has been long standing and frequent may respond slower to treatment due to the fact that significant degeneration may have taken place in various areas of the chewing apparatus. However, it is important to note that even patients with significant degeneration in the jaw joints can often be treated without continuous drugs and without surgery on the joint.

Besides knowing when and how the problem started, the doctor must know exactly where pain is present and what type of pain is present because it is not uncommon for patients to have more than one type of headache. For example, individuals may have a dull ache in the area of the temple or over the temporomandibular joints, which is completely different from a migraine type of a headache that is a pounding, throbbing headache that only occurs once or twice a month. Some patients may have pain which radiates from the back of the neck over toward the forehead, as opposed to pain which is located in the area of the sinus.

Very often, when two types of headaches are present, they require separate treatment, even though they may be interrelated. It is interesting to note that often migraine headaches, even though they are related to a problem in body chemistry, can be aggravated and increased in frequency by muscular headaches related to problems in the function of the jaws. Thus, elimination of TM dysfunction-related headaches may significantly reduce or eliminate even classic migraine-type headache problems. The exact cause and relationship of this is unknown at the present time; however, many professionals in this field have seen it occur for their patients. (Perhaps the stress of a jaw imbalance triggers the migraine?)

As the history interview continues, the examiner will also want to know all of the various symptoms that the patient has. TM dysfunction has been called "The Great Imposter" because symptoms such as pain in the neck or lower back, tingling of the fingers, disturbances in vision, and ringing in the ears all may be related to dysfunctions of the temporomandibular apparatus. On the other hand, they may signal a different type of problem. Only by gathering as much information as possible and correlating the different symptoms, along with a medical history, can the examining clinician begin to develop a diagnosis for the patient.

It is extremely important for you to be as honest and as detailed as possible in your descriptions, even though you may feel that the symptom you are describing could not possibly be related to your headache problem. Be aware that the examiner is very much like a detective and remember that no small shred of evidence is insignificant.

An important aspect of this initial patient history interview is the discussion of the other practitioners the patient has seen for this problem or related problems. The type of tests or diagnostic procedures that were undertaken, the type and duration of treatment, and, most importantly, whether the treatment was successful in any way, all influence the current diagnosis. It is not unusual for patients to achieve partial relief from various procedures, indicating that the particular treatment might be reapplied in conjunction with other treatments to provide an even greater degree of relief. The examining clinician will often request that the patient sign a release so that this vitally important information can be gathered about the previous tests and treatment given.

There are a number of medical conditions which can greatly aggravate problems associated with temporomandibular dysfunction. For example, thyroid problems can affect the irritability of muscles which can lead to an increase in painful spasms in the muscles of the head and neck. Imbalances in hormone levels can also lead to the same situation. This is why many women tend to have headache problems associated with their monthly cycle. Metabolic problems, such as rheumatoid arthritis, can also have significant effects on the temporomandibular joints and therefore, influence headache pain. Moreover, it is important for the clinician to know any other medical problems that the patient may have, since it could create a situation that would mimic a TM dysfunction-type headache.

Very often, the clinician will ask questions concerning the patient's lifestyle. The consumption of caffeine, for instance, will irritate muscles, creating an increased tendency toward spasm and, therefore, acting as a trigger mechanism for headache pain. The same caffeine may also have an influence on the blood vessels of the brain causing caffeine headaches when the daily supply of caffeine is altered. The stress level in the patient's life is also a significant contributing factor to these types of headaches, although often not the root cause, and should be discussed with the doctor who is examining the patient. Again, it is important to be as thorough as possible during this discussion with the doctor.

Depending on the nature and extent of the problems associated with the headaches, the examiner may pursue more varied areas of questioning. Because of the complexity of TM dysfunction and its role as "The Great Imposter," the more information provided to the examiner, the better. Often, in my own practice, I will ask individuals to write a narrative or story about their problems. This gives me the needed information in their own writing, which I then use for my future reference. After the history is complete, the examination can begin.

MOVEMENT PATTERNS
The movement patterns of the jaw can reveal a great deal about the health of the chewing mechanism. For example, a normal jaw should open approximately forty-five to fifty-five millimeters. An opening of between thirty-five and forty-five millimeters would be considered slightly limited but still within an acceptable range.

However, an opening of less than thirty-five millimeters is considered limited and indicates either significant problems within the temporomandibular joint itself or the presence of a significant muscle spasm. (Measurements are relative to the bone structure and size of the individual. One easy "self test" consists of making a fist with the left hand and then trying to put three knuckles between your front teeth with your mouth wide open. (See Figure 3.1) If this cannot be done, there is a strong possibility that at least some muscle spasm is present and, at worst, there is actual damage within the jaw joint.

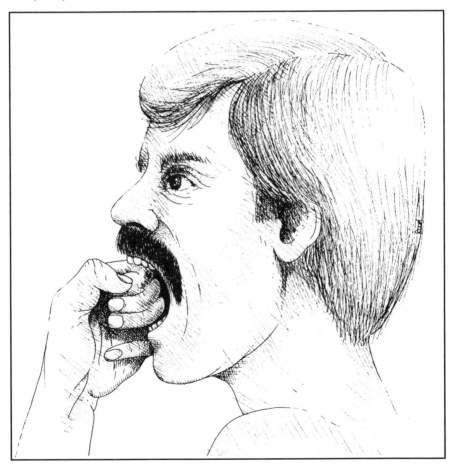

Figure 3.1

Very often, a dentist trained in treating TM dysfunction can tell whether the problem is within the joint or within the muscle by gently pressing on the lower jaw at maximum opening. If the lower jaw opens slightly more with continuous gentle pressure, then muscle spasm is a likely problem. If there is no movement whatsoever then, more than likely, there is a mechanical obstruction within the joint. (You can try this yourself.)

In addition to vertical movements, the path taken by the jaw as it opens and closes can be important. For example, if the lower jaw opens but deviates strongly to one side, the doctor would be suspicious that the joint on the side toward which the jaw deviates is locking or restricted. (However, a muscle could also be in spasm on that particular side.) Very often, the pattern of opening and closing will be erratic. Again, depending on the pattern of erratic movement, this could indicate obstructions within the joints or problems with muscle contraction on opening and closing.

The distance to which the lower jaw can move to the left or to the right is also very useful in diagnosing these types of problems. For example, if the lower jaw moves to one side but will not move to the other side, that is a strong indication that there is a mechanical lock within one of the joints. This type of test is often used to determine whether the problem is actually a locked joint or just a muscle spasm. If a muscle spasm is present, then the jaw movement is limited when opening but can usually move freely from side-to-side. However, when there is a mechanical obstruction in the joint, the opening and closing movement and the movement from side-to-side will be limited.

Many patients mistakenly believe they have a locked joint because they are unable to open, when the problem is mainly muscles which are in spasm. The side-to-side test is a very useful way of determining whether the joint is locked or not. The study of movement patterns has become very sophisticated in recent years. There are a number of companies that have even produced sensing devices connected to computers to measure jaw movement patterns and muscle electrical activity. This particular instrumentation holds a great deal of promise. However, at the present time, there is a significant amount of controversy over this technique. With time and testing, this method of assessing jaw movements may become more and more important in the management of jaw function problems. (See Chapter 2, Figure 2.6)

CLICKING, GRINDING AND SANDPAPER JOINTS

Sounds coming from the joints can tell us a great deal about what is happening within the joints. As mentioned previously, there are even sophisticated sonar devices being developed and hooked up to computers to measure joint noises in the same way that voice patterns are being analyzed. At the present time, this type of sound measurement is in the research stage. However, some day sound may prove very useful in analyzing joint noises.

Currently, the most common method of evaluating joint sounds is with the use of a stethoscope or merely placing ones fingers directly over the joint or at the bottom of the lower jaw in order to feel the vibrations produced from the damaged or misplaced surfaces within the joint. There are many different sounds that can be produced by the disc. The skilled practitioner will be able to differentiate between the many possible types and develop an appropriate diagnosis. However, for the information of the reader, there are a number of easily recognized sounds which can mean trouble. First of all, the classic click within the jaw joint indicates, as we mentioned in Chapter 2, that the disc has moved out of place. The wider the patient must open before the click occurs, the greater damage within the joints because the ligaments surrounding the joints have been stretched significantly. (This makes correction of the clicking joint more and more difficult.)

Joints also make grinding sounds which occur when arthritic degeneration has developed, making the joint surfaces irregular. Some joints even make a loud sandpaper sound which comes from the deposition of crystals due to gout. Many joints will make soft rumpling sounds which are nothing more than slight irregularities in joint surfaces and are nothing to be alarmed about. If, when you chew, your jaws make any sounds which you can hear, it would be wise to have the joints evaluated by someone skilled in this area of dentistry.

TENDER JOINTS

It is extremely important to determine whether the pain is primarily coming from the jaw joints or from the surrounding muscles, because treatment of the problem must be directed at the source (either joints or muscles). In order to determine this, the doctor will perform a test which you can perform yourself. He will place his fingers directly over the joints on either side and press firmly inward. This pressure against the joints normally should not be painful. However, in the presence of inflammation and swelling, joints will be sore or even extremely tender. The doctor will often place his fingers behind the joints or even in the ears to determine if the pressure is built up in that direction also. Some clinicians feel that they can also determine how far a joint is out of position by feeling the pressure within the ear as the patient closes. This has some usefulness; however, it needs to be combined with accurate x-rays and other diagnostic materials, since there is a great deal of inaccuracy associated with it.

Tender or painful joints may mean that only the ligament surrounding the joint is slightly irritated, which is not terribly serious. However, it also may indicate (especially if the pain is severe) that there is significant fluid build-up within the joint or even that arthritic degeneration has begun. *It is very important for you to see your dentist immediately if you press on the joints and feel significant tenderness. Failure to do so could result in irreparable damage to the joints in a relatively short period of time.*

POKING MUSCLES

Most patients either really love or truly hate this part of the examination because, in order to determine which muscles are not functioning properly and which ones are causing pain, it is necessary to do what we call *palpation*. Palpation is nothing more than a firm pressing or massaging of the muscles involved in chewing and supporting the head and neck to determine whether painful knots or trigger points are present. As you can imagine, if a muscle is in significant spasm, this can be quite uncomfortable. Moreover, it is often necessary to press sufficiently hard on the muscle to determine if that muscle is referring or sending pain to another area. On the other hand, if the muscle is not tender or only slightly so, the massaging and pressing motion can be quite comfortable and patients often say, "Don't stop; it feels great."

Since seventy percent of headache pain has a strong muscular component, this part of the examination is extremely critical. Locating the painful muscles can provide the basis for a game plan directed toward relaxing those particular problem areas. It is also important so that as treatment progresses, the success of the therapy can be determined by reduction in pain due to relaxation of the various muscle groups. A failure of relaxation does not necessarily mean that treatment has failed, however, it may mean that a different approach may be necessary.

THE TEETH

The teeth and bite, or how the teeth fit together, is usually one of the last things that is evaluated by the skilled clinician. One important reason for this is that it allows the clinician to avoid jumping to a premature conclusion. It is very easy to look at a very bad set of teeth and immediately assume that they are prime causative factors for the pain that the patient is feeling. However, after working with these types of problems for a while, the doctor soon learns that teeth are only a part of the whole picture and that premature conclusions can be misleading.

Nevertheless, when the teeth are finally evaluated, several important observations need to be made. For example, when the upper teeth overlap and hide the lower teeth, there is a *deep bite* present. On the other hand, when there is no overlap between the front and lower teeth and, instead, a space present, there is an *open bite*. Both conditions can have significant effects upon the jaw joints, causing damage and pain.

In addition, when the front teeth stick out beyond the lower teeth, that is called *overjet*. (The official terminology for this is a Class II bite, a Class I bite being normal.) When the lower jaw protrudes beyond the upper jaw, this condition is often referred to as an *under bite*. (An under bite is termed a Class III bite.) Both conditions can have significant effects upon the temporomadibular joints or the chewing muscles. In examining the teeth, the doctor will observe the gearing of the back teeth together. He or she will also be very observant regarding the amount of wear on the teeth.

Diagnosing TM dysfunction is truly like a detective trying to unravel a mystery: the foot prints or wear patterns on the teeth can tell the doctor a great deal about where the force is being applied between the two jaws and, therefore, against the joints and muscles. Other tell-tail signs can be loose teeth, tender or sensitive teeth, and loss of gum tissue around certain teeth or groups of teeth. All these symptoms indicate patterns of overloading. For example, excessive wear of the back teeth indicates that your teeth are hitting too hard in that area and that the lower jaw is teeter-tottering around the back molars, thereby creating a great deal of damage by pulling the joint out of the socket. (Ouch!)

THERE IS STILL MORE
Since TM dysfunction has been called the great imposter, it is important to make sure that it is in fact an imposter, not a phantom. It is very important that the doctor, therefore, rule out other diseases. To do so, he or she will very often check out movement patterns of the head and neck to determine if there are restrictions

present or muscle spasm. The doctor will als
and the nose to see if there is any disease
possibly do a quick neurological exam.
disease is present in addition to or instea
or she will have a team of competent medical doc
specialties such as neurology; ear, nose, and throat; physiatıy
muscle function specialist); and psychiatry available for help.

DIAGNOSTIC X-RAYS

Temporomandibular dysfunction or disorders have been termed
the disease of the 80's, since it has only been in recent years that
many clinicians have begun treating these problems. One reason
for this is that good diagnostic x-rays just recently have become
routinely available to the practicing clinician. Your doctor may
request one or more of the following x-rays to determine if there
is a TM dysfunction problem present.

> <u>Panoramic X-ray</u>. This x-ray helps determine if
> there are growths or problems within the teeth,
> sinuses, etc. They are not useful in determining
> actual damage in the joint. However, some
> doctors will use them as an initial x-ray.

> <u>Transcranial X-ray</u>. Transcranial x-rays have
> been used for a number of years to determine
> joint position and disease. They can be useful in
> helping the doctor determine the proper course
> of treatment.

> <u>Corrected Tomographic X-ray</u>. These are spe-
> cialized x-rays which require fairly sophisticated
> equipment and yield a great deal of very accu-
> rate information on the position and condition
> of the joint. Many clinicians feel these x-rays are

the ideal special x-ray to be used for the average jaw dysfunction patient. Unfortunately, they are not available in many areas of the country.

C.A.T. Scan. C.A.T. stands for Computer Aided Tomography. This is a special computerized x-ray which is taken at the hospital and is used for determining the shape and condition of parts within the joint. A C.A.T. Scan can be extremely useful in determining the conditions within the joint. However, because of cost, sophistication, and higher levels of radiation, C.A.T. Scans are usually reserved for those patients with the most serious problems.

Arthrography. Arthrography is a specialized technique used to determine the condition of the joint, especially the position of the disc within the joint. Arthrography utilizes the injection of dye into the joint which can be seen on an x-ray. The process tends to be somewhat uncomfortable but yields a great deal of data about the position of the disc. Again, because it is relatively sophisticated and also is uncomfortable for the patient, it is usually reserved for those patients who have a severe problem, often a problem which does not respond to initial therapy attempts. Many doctors use this as an x-ray just prior to surgery on the joints in order to determine the extent of damage.

M.R.I. Scanning. M.R.I. scanning stands for Magnetic Resonance Imaging, a space-aged technology whereby a large electro-magnetic coil is used to align the hydrogen atoms of the water molecules within the body producing fields which can be read by a computer. It is an absolutely amazing technique which provides unbelievably accurate anatomic views. At the present time, it is primarily in the research stage with regard to jaw joint problems, since there are some technical difficulties which need to be overcome to provide accuracy for routine use. In addition, the cost of this type of evaluation is also expensive and, therefore, limits use to the more severe problems.

Your doctor may choose to use one or more of these imaging techniques in order to determine the full extent of problems within the temporomandibular joint. If you have any questions concerning the results, I would not hesitate to request that he or she sit down with you and go over the findings. All of these techniques can be very helpful in determining the extent of joint involvement in a patient with headache pain.

DIAGNOSTIC CASTS

Since many problems involving the temporomandibular joints and the surrounding musculature have their root cause within the gearing of the teeth, it is customary to make molds and fabricate plaster models of the patient's teeth. Often , these models are placed on a machine called an *articulator*, which simulates jaw movements. The reasoning behind this is that most patients who have pain also have muscles which are under spasm. When muscles are under spasm, they tend to pull the jaw out of position, creating a false bite. The articulator is a means by which jaw movements can be analyzed without the distracting effect of the painful muscles. It also provides a method of determining where the teeth fit at the beginning of treatment compared to how the teeth fit after the muscles have relaxed and the joints are no longer swollen and irritated. Many times, these two jaw positions can be quite different. The articulator can be used to determine the amount and rate of change which has occurred. Models which have been mounted on an articulator can be extremely useful in determining a proper course of treatment.

THE DIAGNOSTIC PHASE OF TREATMENT

Because of the complexity in TM dysfunction and facial pain problems, even after extensive history, examination, and diagnostic procedures, the doctor may still only come up with a tentative diagnosis. This will mean he or she has a fairly good idea of what the problem is; however, the doctor does need to test the findings. One way of doing this is through the diagnostic phase of therapy. This usually consists of placing a plastic plate or a soft rubber plate between the teeth and monitoring the patient's response. This phase of treatment will be discussed later in the chapter entitled "Ending The Pain: Treatment of TM Dysfunction." However, this phase is also diagnostic and, in some instances, also provides a further test for a possible diagnosis.

CONCLUSION

You may have suffered headache pain for years because TM dysfunction is a very complex problem to diagnose. It is the "great imposter" which can mimic many types of dental and medical problems such as toothaches, sinus, migraine, ear disease and neck problems. However, with the new knowledge in this field, you do not need to live with pain. If you have a TM dysfunction, you can be helped!

It is time for an examination or a re-examination to confirm your suspicion. This examination must be thorough and complete, with information from as many sources as possible. With this knowledge and the techniques to be presented in the next chapter, your face, head or neck pain may be greatly reduced or gone forever.

CHAPTER 4

Ending The Pain: Treatment of TM Dysfunction

"But I already have a splint and it hasn't helped very much," said Lenore, who had been referred to my office by her dentist. Lenore's dentist had made her a plastic appliance, often called a splint or orthotic, which fits over the teeth so that they cannot come together. Instead, the teeth contact the plastic. She was concerned, since she had already spent a considerable amount of time and money on her first appliance, that I would suggest such a device as part of my treatment.

Lenore's headaches had begun after an accidental blow she had received to the jaw approximately two and one-half years earlier. Shortly after the injury, her jaw began to click and she began to experience severe pain on the left side of her face above, below, and behind her left eye. This problem was aggravated by chewing, talking, and general jaw movements. Her physician had recommended that she see her dentist, who proceeded to fabricate the plastic appliance in order to provide her with some relief. Lenore felt that the appliance had reduced the headaches in frequency and intensity by about one third. However, she was still experiencing a significant amount of pain, although her dentist had repeatedly adjusted the appliance.

Lenore reported that she had originally been wearing the appliance for about twenty hours a day, but for the past few months had only been wearing it eight to twelve hours. At the same time, her consumption of painkillers was on the increase. She was becoming somewhat frustrated and angry because she had been to several physicians, a chiropractor, and her family dentist with only minimal results. Fortunately, after about six weeks of wearing a different type of orthotic device on a twenty-four hour basis, we were able to virtually eliminate Lenore's headaches.

After she had worn the plastic orthotic for approximately six months, it was evident that her teeth would need to be moved using orthodontics in order to place them in a position that would hold the jaw joint in an alignment that would prevent it from becoming inflamed again. Realigning the teeth and having Lenore wear the plastic orthotic at night have allowed her to be without headaches for over five years.

The family dentist who treated Lenore did so with the best of intentions and has helped many patients with the same type of treatment. Unfortunately, Lenore's problem was different. Many people who do not respond to initial attempts at therapy are not hopeless. Unfortunately for them, and possibly for you, the right combination of treatments has not yet been applied.

In Lenore's case, several complicating factors were keeping her from becoming as pain-free as possible. First of all, she needed to wear her orthotic twenty-four hours a day, including eating. In addition, the click in the jaw joint indicated that the appliance needed to be modified in order to move the lower jaw slightly to that it would be in a better relationship to the slipping ore had a number of trigger areas in her facial eeded treatment in order to prevent the pain from all these factors were addressed and treated,

Lenore became relatively pain-free. In this chapter, we will discuss many of the therapies now being used to treat TM dysfunction.

DRUG THERAPIES

Because TM disorders usually involve either muscle spasm or inflammation of the joints, both of which create pain, muscle relaxant drugs, drugs which reduce inflammation, and painkillers are often prescribed for this type of problem. This is especially true if the problem has been mislabeled as a muscle contraction headache. In such cases, the symptom, which is the muscle contraction, is treated with the muscle relaxing drug while the underlying functional problem remains. Many of the headache clinics which have developed around the country tend to rely quite heavily upon therapies based on a particular drug or combination of drugs. Very often, their results can be quite good; but since the underlying cause has not been corrected, continuous drug therapy is needed or, at best, periodically needs to be reinstituted in order to keep the symptoms from recurring. Needless to say, the long-term use of strong medications should be avoided if at all possible.

Fortunately, dentists who are dealing with TM disorders by correcting the underlying problems find the necessity for drugs is greatly reduced. In fact, most dentists feel drugs should only be used in those situations where the pain or inflammation is so intense that immediate relief becomes mandatory. It is important to note, especially with painkillers, that if the pain is caused by a severe muscle spasm due to irritable muscles, it is not uncommon to find even very strong painkillers to be ineffective. There seems to be a protective override mechanism in the body which will not allow this type of pain to be blocked. In addition, with this type of pain, if the muscles are in severe spasm, even very strong muscle relaxants may not be effective. Fortunately, there are ways of relieving these problems without heavy drug usage. We will discuss these ways as we proceed further through the chapter.

SPLINTS (REPOSITIONING ORTHOTICS)

The most common treatment for temporomandibular disorders is the use of *repositioning orthotics,* commonly called *splints.* These devices can be made from a number of different materials and are fabricated in a number of different shapes, forms, and sizes. Splints may fit on the upper teeth or the lower teeth or rest loosely in between the teeth. There are more than a dozen different types of orthotics which can be used. However, they all share the following goals, to various degrees, in common:

> Realigning the Joint. By placing a piece of plastic which is fabricated to fit over either the upper or lower teeth and creating indentations into which the opposing set of teeth can fit, the skilled clinician is able to guide the patient's lower jaw gently into a new position every time it closes. (See Figures 4.1 and 4.2. In Figure 4.1, the lower jaw is out of position creating a displacement of the disc between the two bones. In Figure 4.2, a plastic splint has repositioned the jaw in order to bring it into better alignment with the disc, thus eliminating clicking and often times reducing inflammation within the joint.

> Muscle Relaxation. By placing a plastic plate over one set of teeth, the protective signals traveling from the roots of the teeth to the brain and then to the facial muscles are interrupted. By further shaping the plastic plate so that one side is very smooth, the natural locking together of the teeth is eliminated and the muscles are no longer able to put excessive stress on the joints or upon each other, again reducing muscle strain. (See Figure 4.2)

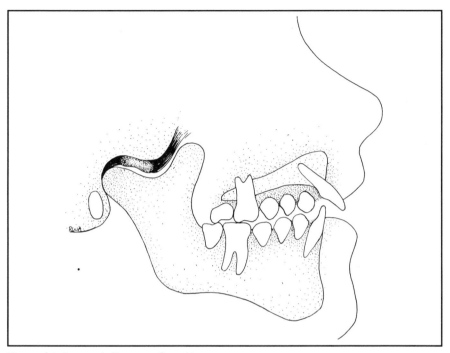

Figure 4.1: Jaw and disc out of position

Moreover, by slightly moving the jaws apart with the use of this plastic appliance, the muscles are stretched and a natural relaxation tends to take place. In situations where there are significant discrepancies between jaw position or tooth position so that normal chewing creates teeth which bang together, fabricating this plastic splint can allow the dentist to create an ideal bite which is much more kind to both the jaw joint and the muscle structure.

Postural Change. Since the lower jaw is attached to the base of the skull by ligaments and muscles, guiding the jaw into a new position will create contraction or stretch in these muscles.

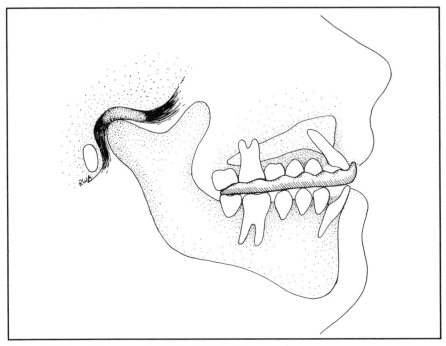

Figure 4.2: Repositioning orthotic (splint) in place

Always remember, that when the length of a muscle changes, it will affect all the surrounding muscles. To show the effect of changing the position of the lower jaw and, therefore, the surrounding muscles, try a simple experiment. Jut your lower jaw forward as far as possible and then move your head back over your spine. Notice how the tension in the muscles under your chin relaxes. Next, move both the head and the jaw forward. This creates a great deal of discomfort in the submandibular, or muscles under the jaw. By moving the lower jaw, the skilled clinician can affect, the posture of the head upon the spinal column, thereby affecting the tension and dynamics of the neck muscles.

Placing an orthotic between the teeth will change the center of gravity of the head, which affects the tension on the facial and neck muscles. This can be very beneficial to patients who have TM dysfunction problems which are aggravated by spastic neck muscles.

Some splints are fabricated out of soft materials; some from a hard plastic; some from a thermoplastic material that allows them to be reshaped after being immersed in warm water. There is even one type that consists of a fluid-filled sac (Aqualizer™) which rests over the biting surfaces of the teeth and cushions the biting surfaces while also performing an automatic leveling function between the left side and right side of the bite.

All of these splints have their place, depending upon the particular problem involved. Please be aware, however, that there is a great deal of controversy over why and when to use what type of splint. Consequently, the experience of the practitioner involved is often the factor which determines which splint is used. Therefore, I will discuss only the more common applications of the more frequently used appliances.

Soft Splints. Soft splints are used mainly in the early phases of treatment. They tend to wear out rather quickly and, in certain instances, can aggravate a clenching habit because their softness still allows one set of teeth to indent and lock into the splint, creating leverage forces (Splints which are made of a very hard material do not allow this locking motion and increase in forces.) There are many factors involved in the choice of soft splints, not the least of which is the amount of muscle spasm, inflammation, or pain present. Usually, patients which are in a very acute or painful stage will be provided with a soft appliance at first. Often, they later will be graduated into a hard appliance.

Hard splints. These orthotics can be divided into a number of different types based on the position in which they hold the lower jaw in relation to the upper jaw. The first hard splint style is called a *flat-splint.* It is basically a piece of plastic which fits over one set of teeth and is completely smooth on the opposite side so that the opposing set of teeth, when in contact, glides freely in any direction. It is one of the gentlest splints used. However, more often than not it is used in the initial phase of therapy in order to achieve relief for the patient.

As therapy proceeds, various slopes will be added to the appliance to more nearly simulate chewing against a normal, opposing set of teeth. As these slopes are added, individuals are gradually acclimatized to chewing against something which has similarities to their original set of teeth. This has the distinct advantage of moving such individuals closer to a point where they can be "weaned" off the appliance. This type of appliance is called a *superior-repositioning appliance* or a *guidance appliance.* The goal of the dentist in this situation is to provide a final appliance with a guide ramp that allows the front teeth to lift the back teeth apart when moving from side to side. This most closely approximates the ideal motion of normal teeth.

Anterior Repositioning Appliance. Indentations are made in this appliance so that as the mouth closes, the lower jaw is guided into a position different from the position it would normally occupy. Very often, the jaw is directed forward in order to move it into a better relationship with the disc, which has slipped out of position. Therefore, initially, it may be necessary to move the jaw quite far forward to achieve this end. With time, however, the plastic plate can be modified to allow gradually the jaw to close farther and farther back toward its original position. If the use of this splint is successful, a clicking joint can be eliminated and healing will take place within the joint. (See Figure 4.2)

Unfortunately, the jaw cannot always be moved completely back into its original position. In such an instance, the teeth will need to be repositioned to hold the jaw in this new relationship. Most practitioners would prefer to move the jaw to a position that is as near its original starting point as possible, since keeping the jaw a significant distance forward holds the possibility of the click returning at a later date. In addition there is difficulty in maintaining the jaw in an extremely forward position over a long period of time.

The above procedure is termed *recapturing the disc.* This procedure creates a significant dilemma for the practitioner. If the disc is successfully recaptured and the jaw can be moved back into a near-normal position, treatment becomes relatively easy. However, if the disc cannot be recaptured and, therefore, the jaw needs to be held significantly forward in order to hold the disc in position, the long-term outlook is not as predictable. The dentist then must decide whether to allow the patient to function without a disc between the two bones or to take measures to hold the patient's jaw forward significantly. Both concepts have their advocates.

However, many practitioners find that even though patients may not have a disc between the two bones, they can be kept comfortable and pain-free, with minimal damage to the joint, by wearing a splint on a part-time basis at night as long as the teeth fit in relatively good alignment or are made to do so by orthodontic means. It must be said, however, that as long as the disc is not too far out of alignment it may be best for the doctor to attempt to recapture the disc rather than leave it out of position. I say this because a disc between the two bones is natural and, therefore, the most healthy construction of the joint.

Pivot splints. These splints are either to reduce the inflammation within the joints, allow the disc to slip back into place, or reduce any tendency toward clenching. The pivot splint is basically any plastic plate, either on the upper or lower set of teeth, which allows only one point on one or two teeth in the opposing set of teeth to contact. If there is significant irritation within the jaw joints, or if an arthritic process has taken place, this type of splint, when applied in a limited manner, will modify pressure within the jaw joint. What is actually happening is that a teeter-totter is created using the molar area as a fulcrum.

The nature of this splint dictates that it should almost never be worn for twenty-four hours per day for any longer than six or seven weeks. However, it can be used as a part-time splint without any problems. Pivot splints can be very effective in reducing clenching, since individuals will be unable to exert significant force on just two teeth. (The protective mechanism in the root structure will not allow this.) Therefore, individuals will tend not to clench or grind their teeth heavily.

Some important thoughts for splint wearers. It is extremely important for you to be aware that successful splint therapy, to a great extent, depends upon the commitment of the patient. Therefore, it is absolutely imperative for you to follow the dentist's instructions to the letter. For example, if a splint is to be worn for twenty-four hours a day, including eating, it must not be taken out for even a few bites of food. To do so might trigger protective reflexes in the muscles which can cause contraction and a return to painful spasm. Even worse, such unprotected chewing could result in tearing of the delicate tissues healing within the joints. On the other hand, if the doctor has recommended that the splint be taken out for certain periods, it is extremely important that the splint be removed at the prescribed time so that proper exercise can be provided to the muscles or to allow for a resettling of the bite. There is an old saying among clinicians that practice this art: You can fool me; you can fool yourself; but you can't fool the jaw joint. If you want to get the most out of your treatment, please do not try to fool anyone. Following instructions is your best chance of success!

CONCLUSION

Pain relief, in the form of splints, come in all shapes and sizes: big ones, little ones, fat ones, thin ones, hard ones, and soft ones. Their use is determined by the type of problem you have. Splints allow the modification of not only the function of the jaws and teeth, but also the function of the head and neck as well. It is truly amazing how such a small piece of acrylic can have such far-reaching effects on such a large group of muscles, thus eliminating all sorts of aches and pains.

As we have seen, splints are not necessarily easy to wear. The disruption of normal chewing patterns and speaking patterns caused by splints requires an adaptation period. However, relief from a life of painful headaches or potential jaw degeneration is usually motivation enough to bear the inconvenience of splints.

In addition to wearing a splint, there are other important ways you can relieve your pain and keep it from returning. Muscles must be relaxed and brought to their optimum state of health. Ligaments and joints must heal and be protected. In the following chapters I will discuss how this–and more–can be accomplished.

CHAPTER 5

Arthritis & Pain: Keeping It Out of Your Head

A close friend of mine named Jim confided to me over lunch that his wife was unable to attend an especially important social gathering, because she had been stricken by a severe migraine headache. I could hear the concern in his voice as he described the increasing frequency of these headaches and the significant disruption of their lives.

Jim knew that a sizeable portion of my practice was dedicated to helping patients with headaches due to jaw function problems. However, he had hesitated to discuss Pam's problem with me since she had previously been diagnosed as having migraines by the family physician. At his request, I agreed to see her later that week.

When Pam arrived in my office, she was in relatively good spirits and complained only of a mild, dull headache which seemed to emanate from her ears. She said, however, that with increasing frequency over a period of hours, the pain would gradually worsen until her whole head was throbbing. Very often she became nauseous. When this occurred, Pam said the only thing she could do

71

was lie flat on her back with a cold towel over her forehead. Then, after a few hours, the pain would begin to subside.

Antihistamines had been prescribed because one physician felt the problem might be related to her sinuses. These provided mild but temporary relief. More recently, after a number of sophisticated tests proved negative, anti-migraine medications were prescribed. Again, this provided only temporary relief. It seemed nothing could stop the pain.

As we discussed Pam's problem further, she reported that when she was younger her jaw would click when she opened and closed her mouth. Occasionally, she noted, she would get headaches. However, as time went on her jaw began to lock. But this and the headaches eventually passed. It was not until recently as she was exposed to more stressful situations that the dull, aching pain appeared with periods of severe headaches. She felt the next stop after my office would have to be a psychiatrist.

When I examined Pam, there was a grating sound coming from both jaw joints, and they were quite tender to the touch. In addition, she had many head and neck muscles that were tender. X-rays confirmed my suspicions. Pam had severe osteoarthritis of both temporomandibular joints. Her muscles were overloaded and sore from trying to protect the joints and at the same time from trying to allow normal jaw movement. Fortunately, we were able to eliminate Pam's headaches without surgery or medication.

A rthritis is a medical term used to describe a large number of degenerative processes involving the joints of the body. In its earliest form, arthritis can be a mild irritation of the joint with very little pain. At its worst, arthritis totally destroys the body joints it affects, bringing with it an unbelievable amount of pain. Not only does the pain come from the joint itself, but it also comes from the surrounding muscle structure which is severely strained by trying to protect and limit the motion of the joints. In this chapter you will learn all about arthritis in the jaw and how you may prevent it.

OSTEOARTHRITIS

Osteoarthritis results from wear and tear on the body's joints. Thus, it is distinguished from rheumatoid arthritis and other similar forms of arthritis which are actual active disease processes caused by malfunctions in the immune system or infection.

Osteoarthritis is one of the most common human afflictions. In fact, osteoarthritis is one of the most common afflictions for all mammals, except bats and opossums. Even whales and porpoises, who spend their lives in a relatively weightless state, swimming the oceans, develop osteoarthritis. This crippling disease even affected pre-historic man, evidenced by bone spurs and degeneration found on fossilized bones.

Osteoarthritis is often assumed to be a disease of old age. This is simply not true. There are many people who reach a very ripe, old age with little or no evidence of osteoarthritis. Conversely, there are many young people who already have a significant amount of damage in their joints. People also assume that osteoarthritis is more common in those people who engage in vigorous, physical activities that would tend to punish their joints. However, again, the reverse is true. Osteoarthritis is actually more common in those people who are not physically active and have sedentary lifestyles.

In the following sections, we will discuss the arthritic process and its direct relationship to the temporomandibular joints and the development of head and neck pain.

THE SPONGE CONCEPT

Before we proceed, let me give some additional background on joints. It is important to recognize that there is a great deal of expansion and contraction in the body's joints. For example, if you were to measure yourself just before going to bed, and then again, immediately upon awakening, you would notice that you had increased in height by approximately one-half to three quarters of an inch. This occurs because the pull of gravity upon your body structures during the day compresses the cushioning surface of each joint. This cushioning surface is called *cartilage*. (See Figure 5.1). Cartilage is very much like a dense sponge which contains many little cells which help to maintain and repair the cartilage structure. Interestingly, cartilage is one of the few tissues in the human body that does not have a blood supply. Consequently, it must rely on nutrition and removal of waste products purely by the movement of molecules through its sponge-like material. Remember, for a sponge to operate effectively it must be compressed to squeeze liquids out and, then, must be allowed to expand for the liquid to move back into the sponge's pores. Since the cartilage in our joints works like a sponge, it is important to apply pressure that compresses the cartilage and forces fluids out along with waste products and alternately allows the cartilage to expand and draw in nutrients. Cartilage is so dense that this expansion and contraction does not occur immediately. For expansion to take place or for compression to occur may require hours.

As an orthodontist who treats a significant number of patients with head and neck pain, I often request that x-rays be taken of the temporomandibular joints and am amazed at how often even young patients develop arthritis within these joints. However, it is not surprising since these particular joints are unique: they can function for twenty-four hours without rest, because some patients clench their jaws and grind their teeth day and night. This prevents the joints from resting and, therefore, stops the cartilage from expanding.

On the other hand, there are many individuals who, because of their jaw structure and a phenomenon I call the *pivot effect* (See Figure 5.2), never achieve pressure within the joint sufficient for compressing the cartilage. Both of these groups seem to exhibit a higher incidence of arthritic degeneration in the temporomandibular joints. So, either by underloading or overloading the joint, the potential exists for a lack of nutrition or an increase in waste product build-up to occur, thereby setting the stage for possible arthritic effects.

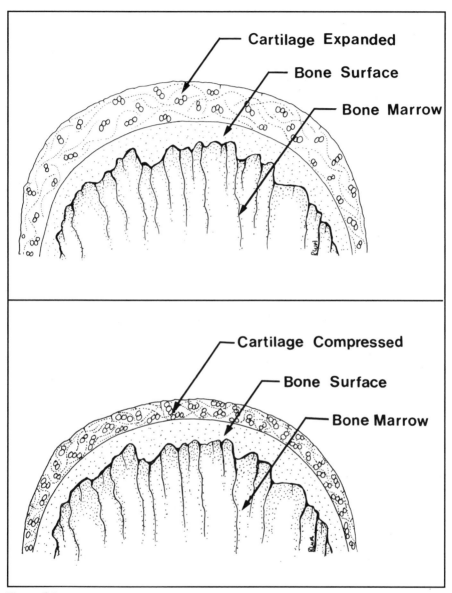

Figure 5.1

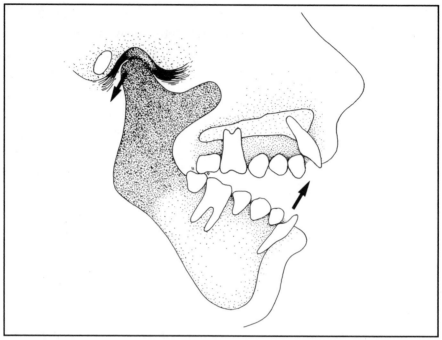

Figure 5.2: Long, thin, verticle facial structure in which back teeth contact first upon closing. This creates a pivot point. As the jaw closes further, the temporomandilar joint is strained.

ARTHRITIS: START TO FINISH

There are still many unknowns about degenerative arthritis and its causes. However, there are some things that are known. For example, one of the first things that occurs in degenerative arthritis is a breakdown in the cartilage covering the surface of the joints. In the case of the temporomandibular joint, the significant area of breakdown would be the cartilage covering the condyle part of the lower jaw and the surface of the joint socket. This breakdown begins when microscopic changes take place in the cartilage, causing it to lose its cushioning effect. Consequently, instead of being smooth and resilient, the cartilage becomes hard and begins to develop cracks. Once it is no longer able to protect the underlying bone, changes in the thickness of that bony layer begin to take place. With time, this bony layer increases considerably in thickness. This is called *sclerosis.* Concurrently, the lining of the joint also will begin to show similar signs of wear and tear.

As the damage increases, inflammation begins to develop and the process progresses more rapidly. Eventually, more bone is added to the inflamed area and the shape of the joint becomes distorted, smooth surfaces become bumpy, and bony projections begin to form. The more inflammation that develops in the joint, the more painful it will become. Unfortunately, the more irregular the joint becomes, the more friction and rubbing will occur, and the more inflammation develops. This becomes a vicious cycle. For this reason, in many individuals the progression of the disease tends to become more rapid as time goes along.

In the early phases of this disease, it is very common for no pain to be present at all. As a matter of fact, I have found significant damage beginning to occur in temporomandibular joints without the patient ever being aware that a problem was present. However, as damage to the joints becomes more pronounced, pain often develops and, thus, people begin seeking medical attention. Unfortunately, significant amounts of irreversible damage may have already occurred to the joints and surrounding structures making long-term management and treatment more difficult.

Usually, this disease is not totally silent. There is almost invariably some signal given to the patient that a problem is developing. This signal may be in the form of a headache or may be in the form of an unusual change in noises occurring within the joints. Therefore, if head, neck pain, or noises begin to develop, it is absolutely imperative that you seek the advice of a trained and knowledgeable professional.

FACIAL STRUCTURE AND ARTHRITIS

The shape and structure of your face will have a direct impact on the forces that are transmitted to the TM joints and this may determine whether or not you are prone to developing arthritis of those joints. Researchers have studied the effects of pressure changes on joints by removing one end of a muscle on the leg of an animal and repositioning it slightly. After a while, the animal will begin to develop arthritis in the joints above and below the repositioned muscle. Because of the new forces present after the muscle is repositioned, certain areas of the joint begin to become overloaded or underloaded, causing microscopic changes which eventually result in arthritic degeneration.

A similar situation can occur in the jaw joint because of the great variation in the structure and shape of the human head. The same structural problems that cause stretching and tearing of the ligaments of the joints also have a significant impact on the development of arthritis in each individual. For instance, Figure 5.2 is an example of a person with a long, narrow face. when this person closes his or her mouth, the first teeth to touch are the large molars in the back. This happens because the shaded portion of this jaw has grown insufficiently. As a result, these molars will become worn out more quickly. In severe cases, these teeth can crack, chip, or even die due to the excessive forces caused by the improper facial structure. However, this is only a small part of the potential problem. When people with such a facial structure attempt to close their lips during swallowing and chewing, their lower jaw is pulled out of its socket, stretching the ligaments and, thereby, loosening the jaw joint. (The condyle is pulled down and back.) There is also the possibility that because of this stretching, the jaw joint will be *underloaded.* That is, there will not be sufficient pressure in the joint during chewing.

As we have discussed, the joint cartilage has sponge-like qualities. Therefore, if the joint is not compressed sufficiently, waste products will not be removed from around the cartilage cells. Moreover, when the cartilage has not been compacted, it cannot later expand, drawing nutrients into itself.

You will recall that cartilage has no direct blood supply; therefore, it must rely on alternate periods of expansion and compression to properly nourish and remove waste products from its component cells. Without this expansion and compression, the net effect is an eventual breakdown and degeneration in the cartilage, thus creating a situation where the body naturally will lay down bone and, thereby, begin the arthritic process. In addition, there is the possibility that, because of inadequate stimulation in this type of facial structure, the necessary mechanical stimulation to produce joint lubricating fluid may also be compromised.

On the other hand, people with a fairly large lower jaw and a square facial profile can suffer from overloading of the jaw joint. These people often have excessive jaw growth as indicated by the shaded area in Figure 5.3. Thus, when such people begin to close their mouths, their front teeth contact first leaving a small gap between the back teeth. As these people close their mouths further, their jaw is naturally pushed back against the front teeth and

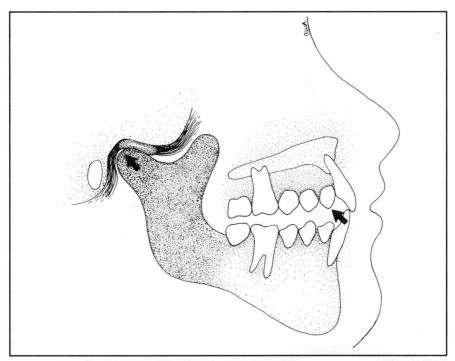

Figure 5.3: Facial structure in which upon closing front teeth touch first. This pushes the lower jaw back and creates strain on the temporomandilar joint.

compression or overloading of the joint may occur. (The condyle is pushed up and back in the socket.) Under such conditions, the cartilage may become overly compressed. This may prevent the cartilage from later expanding and taking in nutritional components for its cells, or the cartilage cells may be injured by this overloading. (If you are a chronic clencher or grinder, your joint never may be relieved of its load. Therefore, the cartilage may never be able to swell and expand, and the cells within the cartilage may die or may be damaged due to a lack of nutrition. In either of these circumstances, the stage is set for breakdown in the protective surface of your joints. Over time, further degeneration can take place in the bony components of the joint, the final result being advanced degenerative arthritis.

It must be emphasized that these problems begin as our faces and heads develop their shape, which means that early damage may be taking place during the teenaged years. Very often, the first signs that a child is developing a problem in this area become evident in the muscle structure. The body has a wonderful protective mechanism whereby the muscles protect the joints from damage. This mechanism is called *splinting* or *tensing-up*. Because of this, one of the first signs that damage is occurring in children can be tiredness of the muscles after chewing or headaches under stress. Muscles which are chronically tight become tired easily and can go into spasm, thus creating headaches.

Fortunately, if children are examined at an early age (four to seven years old), an orthodontist with an appreciation for the mechanics of the temporomandibular joint, along with a knowledge of the growth and development of the head, can do a great deal to redirect the growth of the facial bones so that abnormal joint stresses are minimized and reduced. Occasionally, however, the problem is so severe that only a moderate change can be made and final correction requires surgical repositioning of the jaw bones. We will discuss the correction of such cases in a later chapter.

Beyond the structural considerations of degenerative arthritis, the roles of heredity and diet come into play. Of course, heredity is something we have no control over. However, knowledge of family history with regard to arthritis can prove useful. It can alert people to the fact that they may have a high risk for developing joint problems and, therefore, must take stronger measures to avoid the debilitating effects of degenerative arthritis. If people are not sure of their family history, a few telephone calls and questioning of family members can gather the information relatively quickly.

On the other hand, we do have control over diet. Although we do not know all the answers with regard to the chemical complexity of the arthritic degenerative process, a great deal is beginning to be learned. The fact that Eskimos have very little arthritis points to the possibility of dietary influences. Researchers have found that in countries where higher concentrations of northern cold-water fish are in the diet, the incidence of arthritis and heart disease is markedly reduced. In addition, there are a number of other nutritional steps that can be taken to minimize the impact of this disease. We will discuss this in much greater detail in the chapter entitled: "Vitamins, Minerals & Food."

RHEUMATOID ARTHRITIS

Rheumatoid arthritis is very different from degenerative or osteoarthritis. Rheumatoid arthritis is an autoimmune disease, characterized by the body's immune system attacking the lining of the joint spaces which creates inflammation and eventually degeneration and disfigurement.

Of course, rheumatoid arthritis also attacks the temporomandibular joints. If uncontrolled over a significant period of time, this disease can literally melt away the condyle portion of the lower jaw creating in the anterior of the mouth a significant *open bite* similar to that shown in Figure 5.2. In such cases, the front teeth will no longer touch each other because the lower jaw is becoming shortened by the arthritic process. Fortunately, there are a numbe⁻

of treatments that can be used to slow the progress or even halt the progress of this disease. However, at the present time, there is no known prevention for rheumatoid arthritis.

When rheumatoid arthritis is active and the joints are tender and swollen, significant relief can be given by placing a plastic orthotic plate between the teeth. This treatment is successful in providing relief because rheumatoid arthritis often creates a significant improper positioning of the jaw bones, which in turn places greater strain on the muscles, creating a potential for muscle spasm and headache pain. By placing a splint between the patient's teeth, significant relief can be given to the overloaded muscles, thus reducing headaches. Unfortunately, this, in and of itself, does little to reduce the damage rheumatoid arthritis causes to the temporo-mandibular joints.

Adequate treatment of this disease requires significant medical intervention by the patient's physician in the form of drug therapies. However, the good news is that a great deal can be done to halt the process. Once the inflammation has gone out of the joints, it is possible to surgically reposition the jaws and, thereby, rebuild the normal relationship that the patient once had within the jaw structure. This can create a harmonious facial appearance, a more relaxed muscle structure, and more ideal forces within the already damaged temporomandibular joints.

PSORIATIC ARTHRITIS

Arthritis due to an attack of psoriasis adds more discomfort upon an already discomforting disease. The pain and aggravation which accompany psoriasis are bad enough without involvement of the joints. However, it is even greater problem when the temporo-mandibular joint is affected.

As with rheumatoid arthritis, medical intervention is the only way
ty against psoriatic arthritis. However, since muscles
stress in protecting the joints and compensating for
ure, a plastic splint orthotic can go a long way to

reduce a patient's discomfort. Very often this, along with adequate medical treatment, can significantly reduce the debilitating effects of this disease.

GOUTY ARTHRITIS

In centuries past, gout was once thought to be only a disease of the rich. However, it is now recognized to be related to a chemical defect within the patient's body chemistry which causes the excessive precipitation of uric acid crystals within the joint spaces. These crystals are almost like grains of sand and, as you can imagine, will produce significant discomfort when they are inside a joint, especially the temporomandibular joint.

It is interesting to note that this particular type of arthritis produces a sound within the joints which is unique. Most arthritic processes create sounds in the joint as though there is friction or rubbing or crinkling of paper. With a joint that has been filled with uric acid crystals, the sound becomes very much as though pieces of sandpaper were being rubbed together. One of my patients described it as: "A distinctive and unpleasant sound indeed."

Medications and changes in the diet can do a great deal to reduce or eliminate the uric acid crystal formation within the joint spaces. Along with this, corrective action can then be taken to reduce stress on the muscle structure and compensate for jaw positioning problems. This is done with the use of orthotics and physical therapy. Fortunately, in this instance, a great deal can be done to provide relief and comfort for the patient.

CONCLUSION

We have discussed some of the different arthritic processes which can affect all of our body's joints. In the case of degenerative osteoarthritis, a possible mechanism for the development of this disease and its relationship to facial structure was demonstrated. My good friend's wife, Pam, had a fairly narrow facial structure, thereby creating a situation of underloading and stretching in her temporomandibular joints. Over the years, the problem progressed and headaches developed. We were able to give her relief by first accurately diagnosing the cause of the problem and, then, providing her with an appropriately designed orthotic, supplemented by aggressive physical therapy to eliminate trigger points and provide blood flow and relaxation of muscles. Unfortunately, Pam's jaw structure was "off" to such a significant degree that it was necessary, in order to stabilize the joint in the proper position, to surgically reposition the jaw bones and orthodontically move teeth. However, her relief was dramatic and has lasted. She feels the results were well worth the effort. Like Pam, if you have headaches and your jaw makes noise, relief is possible. But it is important to seek help before your TM joints are severely damaged making treatment more difficult.

In addition to mechanical and medical therapies, the role of nutrition has been mentioned. We will explore how you can make a major difference in your headache pain through diet in chapter 9. How to prevent this from happening to your children will be discussed in chapter 11 "Children Can Be Headaches: But They Shouldn't Have Them."

CHAPTER 6

Physical Therapy and Other Methods of Relief

Carol had come to my office complaining of severe headaches which she said varied from a dull ache around the eyes to an intensity that caused her entire face to hurt. She reported the pain felt like a tight steel band that was clamping tighter and tighter around her head. When she first arrived in the office, she was really feeling quite terrible. However, within just a few days after a repositioning orthotic was placed between her teeth, she experienced almost complete relief. Carol thought it was a miracle, and I was certainly excited about her result. Then, a few days later she arrived in the office looking as if she had spent all night out on the town. The minute I saw her, I knew she was in pain and that something had happened to interrupt our excellent progress. Carol said the headaches were back, although not quite as severe as before. The headache started Saturday afternoon and continued through Sunday. This was Monday.

Upon examining Carol, I noted that her jaw joints were not making noise, as they had been before we had begun the treatment. I knew, therefore, that the orthotic was holding the joint parts in relatively good alignment. In addition, a number of the muscles within her mouth were not as tender as they had been when I originally examined her. However, upon examining the muscles of her neck and some of the chewing muscles in her face, I noted a lot of tender spots, some of which when pressure was applied, would create shooting pains to different parts of her head. I then asked Carol a few questions, after which I instituted steps which gave her almost immediate relief. While she was in my office, I applied a vapor-coolant spray and gently stretched the muscles. She was then taught how to apply moist heat while stretching the muscles at home. We also arranged for Carol a series of physical therapy visits.

Patrick was a successful salesman for a computer software company who had to do a significant amount of travel for his business. Patrick was now thirty-five years old and had suffered increasingly severe headaches for the past seven years. He had experienced intermittent headaches even before that time. However, it was only within the last seven years that these headaches had been constant and had increased in intensity.

Patrick described two kinds of headaches which occurred simultaneously or at different times. The first headache he described as a sinus headache, below the eyes and just above the teeth. He would often awake with this type of headache and could usually reduce it by taking antihistamines, which he did not like to do since they made him drowsy and, therefore, affected his ability to do his job properly. The other headache occurred right at the top of his head and from there often spread into his neck. This headache occurred mainly when he was traveling. This headache had previously been diagnosed as a stress headache. However, even when he was quite relaxed, he would notice that this kind of headache would still occur.

Both headaches were caused by different structural problems. Patrick had not one but two distinct malfunctions. We were able to eliminate Patrick's sinus-type headache without drugs through the use of a repositioning orthotic. However, the headache which occurred while traveling required a slightly different approach. Physical therapy, muscle stretching, and some modification of habits worked amazingly well and eliminated ninety percent of this kind of headache for Patrick.

I n this chapter, we will discuss the many forms of therapy that can be used, in addition to repositioning orthotics (splints), to help reduce or eliminate the pain and misery you suffer from. Since TM dysfunction is a medical problem with a dental component, many of these therapies are ones which are used by physicians in treating medical problems. Through application in the area of TM dysfunction, these therapies can provide an extremely potent source of relief for patients suffering from this problem. (Carol's case is a classic example of how such therapies can significantly augment the use of orthotics.)

Whenever a patient has a significant flare-up of painful headaches after therapy has been initiated—and we have seemingly been achieving a good result—I always find it useful to back-track. By back-tracking, I mean questioning the patient about the forty-eight hours before the flare-up: what was eaten, where was the patient, in what activities was the patient engaged. It is also important to take into consideration any additional, stressful events which might have increased the patient's overall stress level thereby, tending to aggravate clenching, bruxing, or muscle spasms.

For Carol, the Friday before the flare-up had been relatively insignificant. However, on Saturday morning, there had been a rather significant snowstorm in the area, and Carol decided to shovel the sidewalk. She reported that she had really enjoyed getting out and had had absolutely no problem accomplishing this task.

This episode of shoveling had occurred at approximately 8:30 A.M. By noon, the pain had already begun. Because Carol had considered the weather to be somewhat warm for a snowy winter day, she had dressed a little lighter than usual in anticipation of warming up by shoveling. Unfortunately, Carol made two significant mistakes which will most often adversely affect patients with a chronic tendency toward muscle spasm: (1) she overworked muscles that were not yet ready for that level of activity; (These muscles still had a number of points that were capable of triggering intense muscles spasms. We will discuss trigger points later.) (2) Carol chilled these same muscles thereby activating sensitive trigger points and throwing most of the muscle groups in her neck and facial area into intense spasm. Fortunately, with the application of flourimethane spray and stretching, I was able to give Carol almost immediate relief. I also admonished her to protect those muscles by using scarfs to keep them warm. I also asked her not to engage in any intense physical activity until her muscles were more prepared for it. I assured her, however, that in the long run she would most likely be able to shovel the walk without difficulty.

MORE ON SINUSES
Patrick had two distinctly separate headache patterns with two interrelated but distinct, causative factors. His "sinus headaches" had never really been conclusively identified as sinus headaches. (An aside: There are two distinct types of diagnosis in medicine: *descriptive* and *definitive* diagnosis. A *definitive diagnosis* has hard scientific evidence as its root. For example, an extremely high count of certain types white blood cells would indicate leukemia. The diagnosis would be definitive. However, pain in the area of the sinuses without fever, tenderness, swelling, or any other physical sign is often described as "sinusitis," or a sinus headache for want of a better diagnosis. This is a *descriptive diagnosis* and is prone to be *much more inaccurate.* Unfortunately, many people accept such a diagnosis for life without seeking out a more definitive and positive diagnosis.)

In Patrick's case, the pain in the sinuses was actually referred pain from muscles deep within his oral cavity called the pterygoid muscles. When these muscles are in spasm, they can refer pain, giving the patient the feeling that the pain resides under the eyes in the sinuses. Paradoxically, antihistamines often relieve this type of problem, not because they relieve fluid in the sinuses or drain the sinus itself, but because antihistamines are often mild sedatives which tend to reduce muscle spasm. Antihistamines also have the ability to reduce the effects of the chemical histamine, which tends to be a muscle irritant. Unfortunately, this use of antihistamines is successful in reducing this type of headache but tends to be counter-productive over the long term because the root cause of the problem is not corrected, namely, the spasms of these deep chewing muscles which are often the result of improper dental structural relationships. Fortunately, in Patrick's case, the repositioning orthotic was immediately successful in eliminating the headaches and the need for antihistamines.

The headaches at the top of his head and in his neck, which occurred when Patrick was traveling, were caused by an entirely different structural situation. In driving to make his calls, Patrick would sit for long hours in one position, thereby immobilizing and over-stressing his shoulder and neck muscles, thus triggering muscle spasms. Because these muscles had several irritable muscle fibers called trigger points, which may have developed years ago as a result of several traumatic injuries (either from football or an automobile accident), these muscles were much more susceptible to spasm.

Application of deep heat through the use of ultrasound, along with electronic stimulation of the muscles, provided long-lasting relief for Patrick. (Even though he was still under some stress when traveling to new locations and still had to drive significant distances, eliminating the sore trigger points in the muscles and teaching Patrick how to stretch the neck area during breaks while driving also helped to eliminate the head and neck pain.)

It is not unusual for this type of dramatic result to occur even in patients who have had long-standing headaches. However, often the longer the headaches have been in place, the longer the therapy will take to eradicate them. Fortunately, in many instances the prognosis is very good and treatment can be accomplished without the use of long-term drugs and medication. With this in mind, I would like to discuss the various treatment methods available beyond the use of repositioning orthotics (splints).

COLD APPLICATION AND THE TRIGGER POINT STRETCH

The trigger point stretch is not a new exercise, but a method of relieving painful knots within muscles tissues. Before I describe this useful technique, I think it would be appropriate to explain the concept of trigger points and their significance in the treatment of your TM dysfunction and headache pain.

Shortly before the onset of World War II, the concept of trigger points" was developed by one of our nation's leading physicians, Dr. Janet Travell. The term *trigger point* refers to an extremely painful knot within the muscle which, when stimulated, will refer pain to a distant area of the body. The exact mechanism of the trigger point is not known. It seems that stimulating this muscle knot will transmit an intense barrage of signals to the brain, causing confusion and referral of the pain to another area.

The formation of trigger points seems to occur when a muscle is overloaded or strained, either by an abrupt injury such as the trauma of whiplash or by long-term chronic constriction. This often occurs when neck or facial muscles are strained because of poor posture or a bad bite. When the damage occurs, the affected muscle contracts, but certain groups of muscle fibers fail to relax afterward, remaining "locked" in their contracted position. As you can imagine, after a short period of time, these areas can become quite painful and are somewhat like a mini Charley horse within the

these trigger points act as a mechanism for creating

referred pain and also for increasing the irritability of a muscle. When a muscle contains a number of trigger points, it is sensitized in such a way that it can go into uncontrolled spasm with even the slightest provocation. It is not uncommon for patients to complain of headaches or muscle spasms after spending a short time outside on a cold day and becoming chilled. In addition, increasing the workload of these muscles, often even slightly, can activate trigger points, creating referred pain and muscle spasm. The strain of sitting in one position can also overload muscles containing a significant number of trigger points and, thereby, create referred pain.

It is also interesting to note that there are two types of trigger points: *active* and *passive.* Active trigger points will actively refer pain to another area of the body when pressure is applied for fifteen to twenty seconds. Muscles which contain active trigger points are often painful and become severely painful with even the slightest provocation.

On the other hand, passive or latent trigger points are not actively producing a painful situation. As a matter of fact, it is necessary to look very carefully into a muscle to locate such trigger points. In order for these trigger points to become active and begin to refer pain, it is necessary for the muscle to be significantly overloaded in some way. This overload need not be purely physical, such as overworking a muscle. It can also be due to extremes of temperature or changes in body chemistry, which would tend to aggravate the muscle system.

Due to the cumulative effect of injuries during a lifetime, most people have a number of passive trigger points within their muscles. Of course, because they are passive, people are not currently experiencing pain caused by them. But because of their chronic contraction, passive trigger points tend to shorten the length of a muscle, thereby contributing to the tight, limiting feeling that people experience as they age. It is possible that the reduction of these trigger points may turn back the clock in restoring flexibility, youth, and vigor to our movement patterns.

The prospect of pain reduction and youthfulness are certainly worthy goals, but how does one go about removing trigger points and their effects? The answer to that question is almost too simple: gently stretch the muscle! However, as simple as this sounds, there is a catch. Muscles which contain trigger points, either active or passive, do not want to be stretched. There is a protective response which keeps a painful muscle from moving excessively. Therefore, it is necessary to trick the nervous system into allowing the muscle be stretched. This can be accomplished by the use of a counterirritant. The principal counterirritant used today is cold, such as ice or some type of cold-producing spray. Most practitioners use a product called Spray and Stretch™. When applied to sprayed the muscle, this spray produces a chilling effect which then allows the doctor to stretch the muscle gently.

Once the muscle is stretched, very often almost immediate pain relief takes place. If trigger points have been in place for a long time, it may be necessary to repeat the procedure a few times. It is also important to warm the muscle after the stretching technique in order to increase blood supply.

In some cases, however, trigger points are locked in contraction so tightly that they refuse to let go even after stretching. Under these circumstances, significant relief can be obtained by injecting a small amount of anesthetic directly into the trigger point. Consequently, the muscle will immediately release and the patient will experience relief. Some practitioners have found that placing a needle into these tender spots, without anesthetic, can yield the same results. However, the anesthetic serves to reduce discomfort.

Occasionally, trigger points are eliminated from a muscle only to return within a relatively short period of time. This occurs because there is something that is continually irritating the muscle. This could be a structural problem, a skeletal abnormality, or a bad bite.

On the other hand, this situation could be related to problems with a person's chemistry or level of stress. (See Chapters 7 and 9.) It is important to note that until these problems are corrected, spraying and stretching your trigger points or injecting them with anesthetic will only provide temporary relief!

ACUPUNCTURE
Since we have been discussing the concept of trigger points and the elimination of them by placing a needle within the irritated area, with or without anesthetic, it seems appropriate to discuss acupuncture and its application in the treatment of headaches and muscle problems. The word acupuncture comes from the Latin words *acus*, meaning *needle*, and *pungere*, meaning *to sting*. Acupuncture has been used in China for over 3000 years. It was originally used along with moxibustion, which is the burning of an herb near certain sites on the body. There is an ancient legend about acupuncture which says that this treatment began when a soldier in ancient times was struck by an arrow during a battle. When this occurred, he felt a sensation of numbness in an area of the body far removed from the injury. From then on, by placing needles and studying their results, practitioners developed the art of acupuncture.

Acupuncture theory holds that there are meridians or channels of energy which run the length of the body. These take the form of twelve parallel lines. It is believed that the body's energy flows along these meridians and through the various organs, regulating bodily functions. Along these meridians are approximately 500 specific points which, when a needle is inserted, will affect a major organ of the body. The needles which are used come in a variety of lengths and sizes and are inserted based on a complex number of laws.

There has been much interest and research in the western world on the effects of acupuncture. In a variety of situations, acupuncture does work; and it does so amazingly well. However, as of yet, there is no absolute evidence as to how it works. Various theories have been proposed from direct relationship in the nervous tracks of the body to the release of chemicals from the brain called endorphins, which are natural pain relievers.

Even without knowing how acupuncture works, doctors have seen people undergo major surgeries using acupuncture alone or to have allergies or ulcers cured by acupuncture. Many researchers feel that there is a strong psychological component in the success of acupuncture. Since we are finding more and more connection between the thoughts that people have and actual changes in their body chemistry (psychoneuroimmunology), these opinions may prove to be at least partially accurate.

In the area of migraines, acupuncture has proved useful to some individuals. However, its usefulness in treating the type of headaches we are discussing in this book, namely temporomandibular joint and muscle dysfunction problems, may be more limited, due to the necessity of correcting the structural imbalances which can be the root cause of these problems.

NOTE: At this point, it may be evident to the reader that the placement of acupuncture needles and the needling of trigger points are based on two completely different principles and, therefore, should not to be mistaken as identical treatment. While trigger point therapy is directed to the actual irritation within the muscle, acupuncture relies on a more generalized therapy which is, at this point, not well understood. Again, it should be emphasized that the use of acupuncture for this type of problem may be of limited use and would best be reserved for those situations under which more conventional therapy has not been successful.

HEAT THERAPY

Heat can be an extremely effective method of physical therapy when muscles and tissues are irritated or under spastic contraction.

Heat can be applied in the form of hot towels or a commercially available moist heating pad. These methods allow the heat to be applied over the affected muscle area for a period of twenty minutes to one hour, during which time the heated muscle is periodically and gently stretched. This heat treatment is extremely useful after muscles have been sprayed and stretched or after trigger points have been injected. Heat helps to maintain muscle length and to further reduce muscle spasm. The therapeutic action is achieved through increased blood flow caused by the heat in the affected muscles.

It's important to remember that because of the mechanism of referred pain, the spastic muscle, which contains trigger points, may be in a different location from where the pain is felt. For example, a patient often feels discomfort around the eyes, when the actual source of the painful muscle spasm could be the upper neck or one of the chewing muscles in the cheek. Applying heat or ice around the eyes may provide slight relief but not nearly as much as would the same procedure applied directly to the offending muscle.

DIATHERMY AND ULTRASOUND

Although heat can be extremely useful, often it is necessary to warm the deeper muscle layers more thoroughly. To accomplish this, short-wave diathermy or ultrasound may be used. Shortwave diathermy produces a rapidly alternating electrical current that induces motion in the molecules of the tissues below the body surface. The patient feels a warm sensation which can be a guide to avoid overheating these deeper structures.

Even deeper heat penetration can be achieved through the use of ultrasound. It is the deepest form of heat therapy available and is produced by sound waves which go beyond human hearing and vibrate deep in the tissues, agitating molecules which create heat. There may be other added benefits from ultrasound therapy, since the rapid movement of the molecules may allow adhesions and scar tissue within the muscle structure to be loosened, thereby increasing flexibility.

Ultrasound therapy not only relaxes muscles through the heating process but also makes them less irritable and more flexible by eliminating the trigger points. Ultrasound also can be combined with electrical stimulation by passing both sound waves and a mild electrical current through the same electronic head. The simultaneous application of these two modalities seems to provide many patients with more rapid relief. This happens because the electrical stimulation gently contracts and relaxes the muscle, pumping out toxic waste products that have collected within the muscle due to its chronic tightness. In addition, the mild electrical current seems to reduce the irritability of sensory nerves in the area, thus reducing pain in the muscle. Though effective, ultrasound therapy often requires a few days to achieve maximum benefit because the muscle structures must normalize before healing can take place.

Even though a significant amount of relief can be obtained from relaxing the muscles and stretching them using this type of heat therapy, it is still extremely important to resolve the original structural problem creating the muscular overload. Without doing so, reoccurrence of symptoms is likely. After relief has been obtained and the muscles become more relaxed, it also necessary to maintain a program of actively stretching the muscles in order to maintain their length and avoid further cramping. (In the opening story of this chapter, both Carol and Patrick received benefits from the use of ultrasound therapy, combined with electrical stimulation and a rehabilitative home care program of stretching and exercise.)

E.G.S. (Electrogalvanic Stimulation)

In the previous section, we touched briefly on the concept of using electrical currents to stimulate muscles. This therapeutic method is called *electrogalvanic stimulation* (E.G.S.). E.G.S. works as if you were exercising the muscle without conscious activity. The fact that this exercise is involuntary becomes very important when we realize that muscles that are painfully cramped and under spasm will not voluntarily exercise. By passing a mild electrical current into the muscle, we stimulate the muscle fibers similar to the way the brain would stimulate them through the nervous system. Even though the muscle is in spastic state, passing the gentle electrical current through it will begin to pump the muscle, which increases blood supply and thereby removes toxins which build up during chronic contraction, namely lactic acid (the same chemical that creates sore muscles after vigorous exercise). In a way, the muscles are gently over-fatigued to a point where they will begin to relax.

Electrogalvanic stimulation is accomplished by placing two conducting pads (between two and four inches square) directly over the center of the muscles to be activated. In addition, a much larger six-by-four-inch or six-by-eight-inch pad is used on another area of the body to draw current away. The character of the pulses can be changed from almost a continuous pulse, called *tetany*, to alternating pulses of various intensity and frequency. Even the polarity (the positive and negative poles) can be switched to achieve different therapeutic results. Electrostimulation sessions usually last for between ten and twenty minutes. Initially, one may feel a slight prickling sensation on the skin; however, this usually disappears rapidly.

One of the reasons rapid relief is so common with this type of therapy is that it seems to have an effect on the central nervous system in addition to its effect on the muscles.

I usually order electrical stimulation along with ultrasound therapy for any patient with severe muscle spasm. The results from this type of therapy are very positive indeed. Occasionally, there is a patient who is extremely nervous about the utilization of electronic therapies and, therefore, chooses not to benefit. However, this is rare.

It is unfortunate that ultrasound and electrogalvanic stimulation are not used more frequently. It is amazing how often patients who have been unresponsive to other forms of therapy will find significant relief from ultrasound and especially from electrogalvanic therapy. I hope in the future these particular therapeutic methods will be appreciated more.

MASSAGE

The use of massage for relaxation, and as a remedy for pain, has been around for many hundreds of years. During that time many different types of massage therapies have developed, some of which require the skill of a licensed professional, others which can be used effectively at home. There have been many claims for the curative effects of massage, most of which have been unproven. However, message can be especially useful for sore muscles.

As muscles relax and contract, energy is consumed by oxidizing certain chemicals. This activity produces waste products, chiefly lactic acid, which can be irritating to the muscles. During vigorous activity, the relaxation and contraction of the muscles will cause the heart to beat faster and the lungs to breathe more rapidly. This, in turn, will provide more nutrients in the form of oxygen to the exercising muscles. Normally, lactic acid is carried away in this process and good health of the muscles is maintained.

A problem arises, however, if someone is sedentary. This inactive lifestyle creates muscle fatigue because there is inadequate circulation which results in a poor exchange of nutrients and an inadequate removal of waste products in the muscles. This fatigue can be just as real as fatigue from excessive activity. If the person with a sedentary lifestyle also has a significant amount of emotional tension to deal with, this tension can create chronic muscle contraction without relaxation, causing an excessive build-up of lactic acid. In both instances, it is necessary to exercise the muscles in order to improve circulation and remove toxic waste products.

However, if a person is significantly fatigued, or just plain tired and sore, exercise is not a joyful prospect. Under these circumstances, massage can be very effective.

Massaging the muscles causes waste products to be "milked" out of the tissues while circulation is stimulated. Vigorous massage often produces an increase in respiration and heart rate. Massage also helps relax muscles in spasm, thereby reducing pain. In addition, one of the major benefits of massage is psychological. Since massaging of the body has a soothing effect, deep relaxation can also be achieved.

When used on a regular basis, massage cannot only be beneficial for the person being massaged but also can have very favorable psychological effects on the person providing the massage. It is a wonderful gift which couples can provide to each other. There are a number of excellent books available on massage in any book-store. In addition, a massage therapist can be asked to provide instructions.

As I mentioned earlier, there are many different types of massage available, from a relatively light, stroking massage, to a heavy, deep massage which should be undertaken only by trained profession-als. Heavy deep massage can be very useful and can even reduce trigger points in muscles, restoring muscle length and fluidity. However, it is extremely important when obtaining this type of massage that the credentials of the therapist be examined. Different states have different licensing procedures. In some states anyone can perform massage therapy, while in others a vigorous training program with testing afterwards is required. Improper application of massage techniques can aggravate rather than reduce the patient's head and neck pain. It is, therefore, wise to ask a few questions regarding credentials before beginning. Also please note that if significant trigger point areas exist within a muscle, ordinary massage may aggravate these trigger points, actually making matters worse. Should this occur, a careful examination of all muscles in the area will often reveal trigger points that can be treated, allowing the patient to enjoy massage thereafter.

MANIPULATION

Manipulating the spinal column in order to achieve realignment of structural imbalances in the spine is not without foundation. Chiropractors, osteopaths, and even some physicians are appreciating the use of manipulation in order to realign vertebrae which may have slipped out of position creating an impingement on nerve roots, which is called a *facet syndrome.*

When the vertebrae are out of position, irritation and inflammation can develop which is quite painful and limiting. By manipulating the spinal column, these vertebrae can be repositioned in a way that relieves the pressure.

Stretching of the ligaments holding the spinal column in proper position can occur through an accident, an abrupt motion, or through a chronic posture problem. All of these create stretching and looseness in the ligaments, thereby allowing the vertebrae to slip. When this occurs, muscles in the immediate area will tighten to restrict movement and, after a sufficient time, will become painful due to the build-up of lactic acid. Moreover, trigger points can develop in these muscles. At the same time, adjacent muscles also begin to contract in order to protect the muscles which have become sore due to lactic acid build-up. Thus, a chain reaction occurs. Soon, many muscles are in spasm and the patient has a significant problem. Once the vertebrae have been repositioned, muscle spasm often will begin to lessen immediately. However, if many trigger points have developed in the muscles, repeated manipulation will often not yield lasting relief.

As was discussed in the chapter on arthritis, chronic improper structural relationships may cause overloading of associated joint structures. When this occurs over a significant period of time, arthritic degeneration can occur. This happens in the same way that arthritis was produced in the research animals whose muscles were reattached, creating a structural imbalance in the animals' bodies. Proper alignment, therefore, is extremely important in the spinal column and in the relationship of the lower jaw to the skull. Such alignment avoids painful muscular overload and long-term degeneration.

It is extremely important to consider manipulation in its proper relationship. It can be useful in many cases. However, there are also instances when it may be of no value whatsoever. Manipulation may even be harmful in others. When it is useful, it should not be considered the only treatment, for a TM dysfunction problem. Also, time between adjustments is necessary to allow for ligaments to tighten after manipulation. In addition, muscle strengthening exercises should be undertaken to begin strengthening the muscles which keep the spinal column in proper alignment.

Repeated, forceful manipulation bears the danger of repeated stretching of the ligaments holding the joints in place, thereby making them more prone to slippage. Therefore, the potential for creating a self-perpetuating situation increases, especially in the area of the jaw joint. If the lower jaw is manipulated, it should only be done so in very acute situations where the disc has slipped out of position. Under these conditions, attempting to move the jaw in order to allow the disc to slip back into position can be very useful. However, repeated manipulation can create a loose jaw with a chronically slipping disc.

Manipulation called *cranial manipulation* deals with manipulating the bones of the skull. The theory involved is that the connecting areas of the various bones in the skull, which are called *sutures*, have the ability to move. This movement takes place during what is called respiration, a time when the spinal fluid moves in a pattern around the brain. The theory is that occasionally these bones of the skull will move into mis-alignment, creating a locking and a blocking of proper movement of this spinal fluid. Practitioners providing this type of manipulation call themselves *cranial os-teopaths*, and in some instances have been able to provide relief for patients who were unable to find relief in other ways. Unfortunately, at this point, there is no definitive evidence that this motion of the cranial bones takes place. Even with the most sensitive instruments, it has not been demonstrated. However, since relief is often provided, results may be occurring through a mechanism, which is not yet understood. Perhaps in the future scientific evidence for the usefulness of this type of therapy can be provided.

CONCLUSION

In addition to orthotic repositioning devices, there are a number of other therapies which can be useful in the treatment of your headache pain. At times, these alternative therapies may be overlooked, and, therefore, only drugs or orthotics may be used in order to remedy headache problems. Overlooking these therapies often occurs because the significant role of muscles in pain production is not thoroughly appreciated.

Since heat, cold, ultrasound, E.G.S, physical therapy, and massage are directed at the muscular component of the TM dysfunction problem, they often can be the missing link in providing long-term, drug-free relief. When these modalities are combined with a coordinated program of removing structural problems and rehabilitation, patients can often be provided with more permanent relief.

When the pain is gone, after orthotic wear and reduction of muscle problems, final rehabilitation and stabilization can be accomplished. Teeth may need to be reshaped or repositioned so that they don't irritate muscles or joints. The jaws themselves may even need to be reshaped. There are a number of methods to achieve this. In the next chapter, I will discuss this final step to less pain and better health.

CHAPTER 7
Reducing Stress: and Pain

Laura's headaches began when she was in grade school. They would start early in the afternoon with a dull ache in the area of her temple. Although the pain was not severe, it was enough that she would complain to her mother. Sometimes she would go to bed as soon as she got home from school. Laura's parents had her eyes checked. They were normal. Her parents, then, took her to the family physician, who noted, after talking with Laura, the headaches usually occurred only during the week and rarely on weekends. His diagnosis was: stress headaches. He recommended that Laura relax, not take life so seriously, and use a few aspirin as necessary. However, Laura's headaches continued.

In high school, Laura became more aware that her headaches occurred during times of stress. She was happy to at least be able to reduce the frequency of the headaches by concentrating on relaxing. However, when the headaches did occur, the pain was even more intense and more severe than when she was younger.

Although the "stress headaches" continued while she was attending the local university extension, they were tolerable and not too frequent. However, when she graduated and was about to leave home and begin a new job, the headaches dramatically increased.

The pain became so intense, that Laura found it increasingly difficult to function normally. She felt like someone was jabbing ice picks into both of her temples and driving them deep within her skull behind her eyes. Even worse, strong painkillers had little or no effect on dulling the pain. The only thing that seemed to help was a strong tranquilizer that literally knocked her out of commission. She had numerous medical tests, all of which proved to be normal. The career she had worked for over so many years seemed to be slipping away. She was afraid of losing her job as a result of so many absences. Her life was a disaster, and she was becoming extremely depressed.

When Laura came to my office, she looked pale and drawn. After gathering sufficient information and examining her, I assured her she was not crazy, the fear of which was adding to her stress. I told her she was suffering from a muscle structure which was overloaded due to the poor growth of her lower jaw. Fortunately, with the use of an orthotic, the headaches completely disappeared within two weeks. At the same time, her depression left, her outlook improved, and she became excited about the possibilities of her new career.

You may have been told you have "stress headaches." Many headaches are assumed to be stress headaches or tension headaches because they occur when a person is under psychological stress. Physicians often refer to these headaches as muscle-contraction-type headaches.

Unfortunately, the label "stress headaches" has contributed to the problem of treating this type of headache pain. First of all, when this label is applied, you tend to feel that you may be less then adequate or somewhat abnormal. Often there is an implication that you are slightly crazy or unable to cope as a normal person would. Furthermore, applying this label directs the treatment toward stress alone, without encouraging a further search to determine if other causative factors may be present. For this reason, you and many other unfortunate individuals may go through a lifetime of suffering, feeling that you are somehow inadequate or ill-equipped to handle your daily lives, when, in fact, stress may be only a part of your problem.

Those of us who deal with muscle-related headache problems are becoming more and more aware that although stress can be a prime causative factor in creating headache pain, it often is merely the trigger mechanism which begins a headache. Stress can cause a person to tense muscles of the head and neck which, because they are already overloaded, can go into spasm. Stress is the trigger but the gun powder is an overloaded muscle system. To understand this better, we can look at the diagram of the circle of Figure 7.1-Part A. As we have seen in previous chapters, headache pain can be caused by a temporomandibular joint (J) which is malfunctioning, irritated, or degenerated. As indicated by area B in Figure 7.1-Part B headaches can also be caused by structural problems such as a poor bite, improperly aligned jaws, or even problems with posture. Because of stress (ST), we can contract our muscles sufficiently to make them tired and painful. The diagram represents the interrelationship of all these factors (J-B-ST).

The degree to which each one of these items is a problem often determines whether a headache develops or not. For example in Figure 7.1-Part B, we can see that there is a significant structural problem (B) and a very small amount of stress (ST), but a significant problem within the joints (J). Therefore, the patient may develop a headache. In Figure 7.1-Part C, moreover, without the significant joint problem, the headache probably will not develop. In Figure 7.1-Part D, a significant amount of stress is present while structural and joint problems are minimal. Here again, a headache would develop. However, when the stress is reduced, a headache would no longer be present. It is the relative input of these different parts of the problem which determines whether pain will or will not occur.

When under stress, our bodies often exhibit a number of behaviors which can lead to the painful contraction of already overloaded muscles. One very common behavior is clenching of the teeth during the day or, even worse, during sleep. If this behavior is carried out with muscles that are already chronically

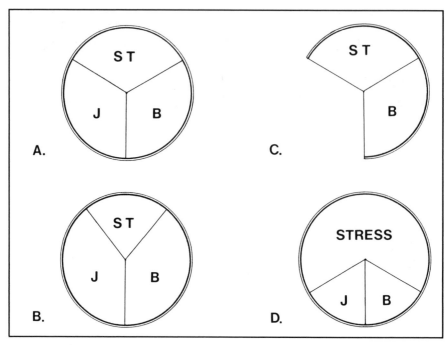

Figure 7.1: ST = Stress, J = Joint, B = Bite

overloaded from trying to protect teeth in a bad bite or by trying to protect an inflamed jaw joint, painful spasm will occur and a headache will result. Many people say: "But the pain is in my forehead, not in my jaw, and you're saying it's my jaw muscles that are in spasm." Because of mechanisms which are not yet well-understood, pain can be referred to other parts of the body. It is as if a short circuit occurs and the brain misinterprets the signal that is being sent. (This often happens during a heart attack when pain is felt in the arm instead of the heart.) The common referral patterns of the head and neck are seen in Figure 7.2.

Another frequent behavior pattern during stress is lifting our shoulders. This seems to be related to the same process that cats exhibit when alarmed: they arch their backs. This behavior, when done with a set of muscles that are already overworked because of bad posture or work habits, will trigger a painful spasm that can refer pain to the top of the head or above the eyes. These are just

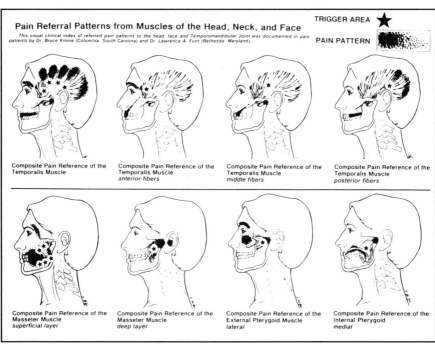

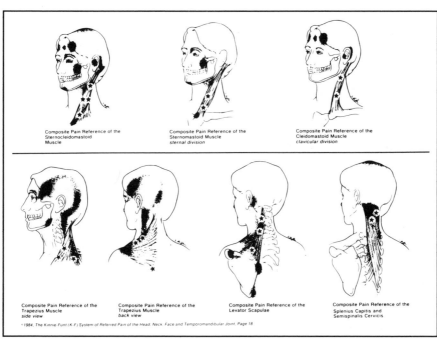

Figure 7.2

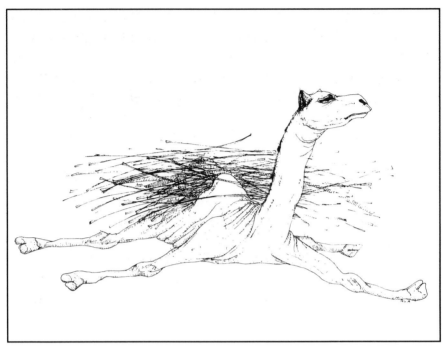

Figure 7.3

a few examples of the way in which stress can overload an already overworked muscle structure and, thereby, create head and neck aches.

An analogy that I have used in explaining the many contributing factors that cause pain is this: Head and neck pain is very much like the camel with straws on its back (See Figure 7.3), each straw being a different factor, such as stress, structural problems, or joint problems. When one or more of the straws is reduced or removed, the pain can often be eliminated. When more of the straw is removed, the camel or patient can function at a higher level of activity and wellness.

DISTRESS

The father of stress research is Dr. Hans Selye. In 1936, Dr. Selye developed the concept of the "fight or flight" response, which is the body's reaction to a source of stress. The term *fight or flight* came from the protective reflex which developed in our species over millions of years of evolution. It is the bodily response which literally prepared our ancient ancestors to either "fight" a wild tiger or run in "flight" from its threat. Below is a list of the various physiological changes that can occur in the fight or flight response:

1. Adrenaline is released from the adrenal glands. The release of adrenaline sets the stage for many of the reactions that follow.

2. Blood sugar increases and fats are released into the blood stream. This provides for quick energy and an increase in strength and endurance.

3. Heart rate increases. This increases the flow of blood to other parts of the body carrying increased nutrition and oxygen.

4. The rate of breathing increases. This provides for increased oxygen to the brain and muscles.

5. Digestion is "shutdown." This reduces blood flow to the intestinal area, thereby allowing more blood for muscle and brain function.

6. Perspiration begins. This helps cool the body which now burns more energy.

7. Blood chemistry changes so that clotting occurs more easily. This is a protective response necessary to reduce any bleeding due to injury.

Millions of years ago, this response proved extremely useful in saving the lives of our ancestors. Today, it can prove useful in situations where immediate action is necessary to save our lives. However, for the most part, today's lions and tigers take the form of unpaid bills, hostile supervisors, and a multitude of other daily complexities. Unfortunately, these tigers are difficult, if not impossible, to attack, and often the opportunity to run is unavailable. Under these circumstances, the chemical changes which take place in our bodies during the stressful response remain in place instead of being burned off by either fighting or fleeing. The problem is this: When these chemicals remain in our systems for long periods of time, significant damage can result.

Dr. Selye developed what he called "the general adaptation syndrome," in which all stressors produced a response which, if maintained, would have significantly damaging effects on the individual. He divided the body's defense system into the following stages:

Alarm Stage. When the individual is exposed to the stressful situation, a number of things occur which constitute the flight or fight response. (See Table 2) One significant effect of the flight or fight response is an increase in the size of the adrenal cortex, which is the outer layer of the adrenal gland.

Resistance Stage. If the stressor remains present and the individual is unable to fight or flee, signs of the alarm stage will gradually disappear. However, residual increases in stress-related hormones will be maintained as the body attempts to maintain its resistance to the stressful situation.

Exhaustion Stage. long-term exposure to the stressful situation will eventually deplete the stores of adaptation energy and the body will no longer be able to cope. Often, the signs of the alarm stage will reappear, possibly becoming irreversible. The final outcome often will result in death due to stress-related factors including exhaustion.

As individuals, we all have specific ways in which our bodies respond to stress. Our particular response is very noticeable when we know where to look. The following is a list of possible signs that we are under stress.

An increase in heart rate	Bruxing, clenching and
A dry mouth	grinding of teeth
Irritability	Sweating
Impulsive or irrational	Frequent urination
behavior	Diarrhea, indigestion,
The urge to cry, run or hide	stomach upsets
Constant fatigue	Hypoconesia (the urge to
An inability to concentrate	move about without reason)
Dizziness	Migraine headaches
Non-specific anxiety (being	Irregular menstrual cycles
fearful, but not knowing	Loss or increase of appetite
of what)	Increased smoking
Feeling wound up, alert	General or specific muscle pain
and tense	Alcohol or drug addiction
Trembling or nervous ticks	Nightmares
Jumpy, easily startled	Neurotic behavior
Nervous laughter	Psychosis
Insomnia	Accident proneness
Stuttering	Increased use of prescribed
	drugs

Any of these signs can signal that we are in a stressful situation which is not being resolved. Unfortunately, the continued production of the stress-related adrenal hormones can have significant detrimental effects on the organs in our body, some of which we are just beginning to understand. Research has implicated constant stress in many of our chronic diseases such as heart disease and cancer, in addition to the more commonly understood ones such as stomach ulcers. When we are in a stressful situation, our bodies are supercharged for action. It is very much like taking our family automobile and pouring nitro-methane dragster fuel in the gas tank. We would get one heck of a quick ride around the neighborhood, and we might even squeal the tires a few times. But continuing to burn that type of fuel in the family car would soon see us taking our last trip—to the junk yard. Unfortunately, constant stress can produce the same effects in our bodies.

DISTRESS VS. EUSTRESS

A very common misconception is that stress is primarily psychological. However, when we think about it, there are many different ways we can stress our bodies. Dr. Selye found very early in his work that stress from different sources—such as physical, chemical, or psychological—produces the same reaction within the body. Input comes to the brain through the cortex signaling that the body is being stressed. These impulses are transferred to an area deep in the brain called the hypothalamus, which, in turn, signals the body to produce the fight or flight response. No matter what type of stress is encountered, once those impulses reach the level of a hypothalamus, the fight or flight response is the same.

For example, if you were to be thrown into a freezing lake in the middle of winter, this would be considered a physical stress. The body would react with increased heart rate and the fight or flight response. On the other hand, if we were to provide you with a strong chemical stimulant or some type of toxic chemical, the body would again react with the same fight or flight response. Of course, psychological stress will produce the same response.

A concept of different types of stress is extremely important because it helps us not to overlook the potentially damaging effects of other stressors beside purely psychological ones. For example, we may be stressed by continually adding chemicals to our bodies such as nicotine or caffeine. (A cup of coffee has the ability to increase the adrenaline level by twenty-five percent or more.) Or, we may be constantly under physical stress due to poor posture, and, especially, poor alignment of the jaws and dental components. These become chronic long-term stressors which can, under the appropriate circumstances, produce the same damaging results as long-term psychological distress.

The net effect of all these stressors is that each one is, again, a straw on the camel's back with the potential for creating degenerative changes in our bodies. In addition, each one has the ability to act as a trigger mechanism for head or neck pain.

Fortunately, Dr. Selye also discovered what he termed *eustress,* which is a good type of psychological stress. This is an extremely important concept, since the difference between eustress and distress is often only a matter of attitude. For example, an excellent skier might find a fairly steep slope somewhat stressing but challenging and exhilarating (eustress). On the other hand, a beginner placed on the same ski run might experience stress that resulted in a feeling of being terrified (distressed). The difference in either situation is the preparation and the thought processes of the people involved. In this situation, it begins to become clear that health has a lot to do with one's attitude; and, fortunately, attitude can be changed.

STRESS AND THE HEADACHE CONNECTION

How then does a person's stress level trigger headaches? To find out, we must go back to our earlier discussions of anatomy, structure, and muscle function. You will remember that the human body has a magnificent protective response which, when teeth are out of position and bumping or the jaw is unnaturally positioned, uses the facial muscles to protect or *splint* the affected parts from further damage. The word splint is used by dental and medical professionals to describe this protective response of the muscles. This splinting response overloads the muscles to the point where they are unable to relax completely. This makes them more prone to painful spasms. A small amount of increased stress is all that is necessary is to trigger a painful spasm when muscles are in this condition.

For example, an individual can go for a long time with head and neck muscles which are chronically tight, due to structural misalignments. When a stressor is added, however, these muscles can be triggered to contract more, and a headache or neckache will occur. The stressor might be a psychological event such as an argument with one's spouse, or a problem at work. Under these circumstances, the added stress may cause the person to slightly tighten his muscles. If the muscles were not already overloaded, this would not be a problem. But when this extra contraction is applied to muscles which are already tense, pain occurs.

Women sometimes get headaches at various times in their monthly cycle because the stressor (the changing hormonal level) tends to increase the tension level of their muscles. If their muscles are already and overloaded, they will go into spasm. (NOTE: It is important to understand in all these situations that stress often acts as a trigger mechanism which would not produce a headache if the muscle structure were not already overloaded and dysfunctional.)

Treatment efforts which are purely directed at eliminating psychological stress, I believe, do an injustice to the patient from the aspect of their total well-being because the underlying physiological causative factors may not have been addressed. These underlying causative factors have the ability to create stress levels of their own, which, over a long period of time, can produce their own set of damaging effects.

DEPRESSION HEADACHES

Stress headaches are often referred to as *depression headaches.* However, research shows that much of the depression patients experience occurs because they feel hopeless and helpless about getting answers and long-lasting relief from their headache problems.

Constant, unremitting pain will cause depression in the best of us. Unfortunately, in trying to help these desperate individuals, some professionals have mistakenly labeled the depression the cause of the problem, rather than an effect of the chronic pain.

Many times, when the headache pain is relieved, the depression goes away. Fortunately, those patients suffering from predominantly depression-caused headache pain are few. It is a tragedy that many people have been branded as depressive personalities because of a misunderstanding of the mechanics in this type of headache problem.

THE RELAXATION RESPONSE

It would take a book to discuss all the possible remedies for reducing the stress level in one's life. Fortunately, there are a significant number of books available in that area that can provide useful information to those patients who would like to remove just one more straw from the camel's back.

Dr. Selye developed what he called the *relaxation response*, which can be extremely useful in reducing the trigger mechanism responsible for initiating headache pain. It also can be helpful in reducing the chronic stress levels which can have such a damaging effect to people's overall good health. The relaxation response is the opposite of the flight and fight response; it occurs when we are perfectly calm, peaceful, and relaxed. There is a lowering of the heart rate, the adrenal glands produce less adrenaline, and the person's overall physiology is relaxed. The trick is to become skilled enough to produce this response within your own body even in the most stressful situations. The only way this can occur is with practice.

The following method can be used to elicit the relaxation response. For the best effect, it should be practiced at least twice daily for the first few weeks and, thereafter, at least once daily. With adequate practice, you will soon notice the ability to relax even under more stressful conditions, thereby producing the therapeutic effects of the relaxation response.

The Relaxation Response

STEP 1: Pick a focus word or short phrase that is firmly rooted in your personal belief system such as relax, let go, etc.. Some people use numbers as a focus of concentration such as one, two, etc..

STEP 2: Sit quietly in a comfortable position.

STEP 3: Close your eyes.

STEP 4: Relax your muscles.

STEP 5: Breathe slowly and naturally. As you do, repeat your focus word or phrase as you exhale.

STEP 6: Assume a passive attitude; don't worry about how well you are doing. When other thoughts come to mind, simply say to yourself, "Oh, well," and gently return to the repetition.

STEP 7: Continue for 10 to 20 minutes.

This exercise is an excellent way to begin reducing stress. However, please remember that to be effective this exercise must be practiced daily! Otherwise, it becomes just another piece of information.

CONCLUSION

We have discussed the role of stress and its relationship to head and neck pain. Unfortunately, treating stress as the root or only cause of muscle contraction headaches has led to people being labeled: depressive, neurotic, or headache-prone. This happens because the underlying structural problems which might exist often are overlooked.

When your muscles are already overworked, or irritable, from a structural problem or a chemical imbalance, (as you will see in chapter 9) psychological tension can then act as a "trigger" to cause muscle spasm and cramping. This can create the deep dull aching pain or the severe tightness around your head and neck.

Remember: you need to correct the structural chemical problems in addition to learning to relax.

In chapters eight and ten, you will learn different methods of correcting misalignments of teeth, jaws and other structures. You will also learn in chapter nine about how chemical problems such as thyroid imbalances or vitamin deficiencies (B12, folic acid, etc.) can irritate muscles and how this can be corrected.

CHAPTER 8

Rehabilitation: Be Healthier and Keep The Pain Away

Frank came into my office one afternoon and said, "You know, Doc, ever since you put this splint in, my teeth haven't fit together very well and the fit is getting worse. When I bite together now, only one tooth touches. I'm glad to get rid of the headaches, but there's no way I can chew without this splint and I don't want to wear it forever." I reminded Frank that when we started using the orthotic, we had discussed the possibility that some type of rehabilitation (stabilization) would be required after the successful completion of therapy.

Since he had been pain-free for a number of months and the lower jaw was no longer changing position from appointment to appointment, I told him that at the next visit we would obtain a new set of diagnostic, plaster models. I told him that based on what I could observe now, orthodontics would be necessary in order to rearrange his teeth so that they would fit again. In addition, I indicated crowns would be required on three of his back teeth. Frank was excited that we could move on with his treatment. Even though he was not thrilled about getting braces, he could see the "light at the end of the tunnel."

The necessity for stabilizing and maintaining procedures following orthotic therapy is very important. The muscle structure must be maintained in its optimum healthy, pain-free state; and teeth must be modified or arranged so they no longer put excessive pressure on the temporomandibular joints or interfere with chewing movements.

If there are significant problems with the alignment of your teeth, one of the main causative factors of your original problem has not been corrected. Therefore, the potential for a recurrence of the original symptoms is high. This, of course, would mean a return to splint therapy and whatever physical therapy might be necessary to again relieve the problem—a situation that could be very discouraging to both you and the doctor. (Occasionally doctors, in their desire to save patients time and money, recommend that rehabilitation and stabilization procedures not be instituted. Unfortunately, this may prove to be false economy in the long run.)

It is extremely important that all options be thoroughly evaluated before discontinuing or limiting splint wear. You should discuss these options very carefully with your doctor, exploring exactly what your options are and what the consequences may be for each option.

EQUILIBRATION: LEVELING THE THREE-LEGGED STOOL

The quickest and easiest method for getting teeth to fit is by reshaping and recontouring the biting surfaces. This procedure is called *equilibration*. The first part of the word is *equal*, which stands for equalizing or leveling the bite. This is exactly what is done. After orthotic splint therapy, one or several teeth may be interfering with proper closure of the jaw. If they are not too large, these interfering areas of the teeth may be reduced and reshaped so that the teeth no longer bump and prevent proper closure. Occasionally, the interference is so small that it can easily be removed in just a couple of seconds. However, most of the time, the interference is more significant; there are a number of teeth interfering. In that case, it is important to have new plaster casts made of the teeth and placed on an articular or jaw simulator where the doctor can "try out" the equilibration on the plaster models first. In this way, he or she can determine exactly where adjustments need to be made, so that neither too little or too much of the tooth surface is removed. Moreover, in those situations where there is a choice of equilibration or a more sophisticated procedure, the doctor can reshape the plaster teeth to determine if equilibration is the best treatment.

Even though equilibration is not as involved as crowning teeth or moving teeth, it is nevertheless a relatively sophisticated procedure which requires a considerable amount of the doctor's time. Therefore, when done properly, this procedure is not inexpensive. However, if by doing an equilibration more expensive and invasive procedures can be avoided, it is certainly the treatment of choice. Even after teeth have been moved with orthodontic braces, equilibration is often necessary in order to adjust the bite further. Both the condition of the biting surface of the teeth and the sensitivity of the patient to changes in the bite have a bearing on whether equilibration will be necessary after orthodontics.

IMPORTANT: Years ago, it was not uncommon to equilibrate a patient's teeth while they were still having pain. This is no longer an acceptable procedure and may actually do more harm than good. When a bite is equilibrated in the presence of pain, the bite may continue to change due to relaxation of muscles or resolution of swelling within the temporomandibular joint. When this occurs, new high spots will appear. Therefore, it was not uncommon years ago for patients to be equilibrated over and over and over again, attempting to provide long-term pain relief. Under most circumstances, irreversible procedures should not be performed (equilibration, crowns, orthodontics) in the presence of significant pain. If you have pain, don't let anyone grind on your teeth!

ONLAYS, CROWNS, AND BRIDGEWORK

If the high spots or interferences in the teeth are too large to be equilibrated without grinding deeply into the tooth, thereby creating sensitivity, crowns or onlays may be used. Conversely, if in order to stabilize the jaw joint teeth need to be made longer or built up, again crowns and onlays may be utilized.

An *onlay* is the *on-laying of a new surface* on top of the tooth. Basically, a new biting surface is created in gold. The tooth's surface usually is prepared by the dentist reshaping it so that it can accept a covering. Onlays are an excellent way of providing changes in the biting surface without removing a great deal of enamel from the tooth's surface.

A *crown,* on the other hand, *covers the entire surface* of the tooth, both the biting surfaces and the sides. It most often is used where large changes in tooth shape or size are needed, or where the tooth previously has had a very large filling. Large fillings tend to weaken teeth, and covering a tooth with a crown will greatly strengthen it. Many times, if there are significant abnormalities in the bite, crowning most, if not all of the teeth, is a possible solution. As you can imagine, this procedure is very expensive and can be quite time consuming. However, the results are usually excellent and long lasting.

OVERLAY PARTIALS AND CAST SPLINTS

Unfortunately, there are situations where crowning the teeth may be unacceptable. Such cases might included: a jaw joint which is continually degenerating due to a disease process or teeth which have significant periodontal (gum) problems and may be lost. Since crowns or onlays are expensive and permanent, their use would not be acceptable under these circumstances. Therefore, a less expensive or temporary alternative, in the form of an overlay partial or splint, can be used.

These devices are basically the same as an orthotic repositioning device (splint). However, they are made of much stronger materials and, therefore, can be made much smaller, covering only the biting surfaces of the teeth. Because overlay partials are often cast in metal or fabricated from ceramic, their cost is considerably higher than a standard orthotic. However, these devices do provide a useful alternative to more permanent and more irreversible procedures and, in many instances, can provide a patient with an appliance which is easier to wear until more permanent changes can be made.

It is extremely important to remember that these appliances are temporary in nature. Nevertheless, they do have the potential for creating changes in the positioning of teeth if they are not monitored frequently by the doctor. Occasionally, patients have arrived in my office after wearing this type of device for a number of years without returning to their doctor. It is discouraging to tell them that what would have been an easy procedure before has become much more complicated, due to the additional tooth movement and build-up necessary to compensate for the changes that have occurred by wearing this appliance without supervision. Needless to say, regular maintenance is extremely important.

GETTING THINGS STRAIGHT: ORTHODONTICS
Of all the methods available for rehabilitating and stabilizing the bite, orthodontics is used quite often. Even in situations where equilibration or onlays and crowns may be necessary, moving the teeth orthodontically often can make a major difference by reducing the amount of tooth structure needed to be removed or reducing the number of crowns required. Orthodontics also can allow teeth to be moved into a position where bridges or crowns can be placed in more ideal positions.

Orthodontic appliances can be limited to just a few teeth or placed on all teeth, depending on the amount of movement necessary. A treatment program can last just a few months or up to two years. Fortunately, there are many new appliances which offer a number of advantages to the patient. There are ceramic or sapphire-type braces which are translucent and take up the natural coloration of the tooth itself, thereby providing a much more pleasing, cosmetic appliance. For those patients who desire the ultimate in cosmetics, lingual or "inside braces" are available. These braces cannot be seen at all. There is a slight disadvantage with this type of brace: speaking becomes more difficult. In general, most patients accommodate this problem quite well after four or five weeks of wear. There are also a number of appliances which tend to increase the speed at which the teeth are moved, thereby reducing treatment time. One of these appliances is even named the "speed appliance," because it has small spring clips which are claimed to distribute force over a longer period of time, thereby increasing comfort and increasing the speed of movement. These advances, plus space-aged metals providing wires which move teeth more rapidly and with less discomfort, provide the patient with an opportunity to have orthodontic appliances for a minimum of time and with a minimum of disruption to their lives.

In many practices, it is not unusual to find patients of all ages being treated for headache problems who subsequently go into some type of orthodontic treatment. We have treated patients from seven to seventy and there is almost no age limit in either direction as long as the teeth are healthy. It is important to remember that many of these patients are undergoing treatment for a better-fitting set of teeth which will support their jaws without strain, rather than for cosmetic reasons. Fortunately, when teeth are well-aligned, they also look good.

THE NEED FOR SURGERY

In the past, a great deal of surgery was done on the temporomandibular joints. But because of improved methods using orthotics, physical therapy, and exercises, now most patients can be helped to a pain-free state without the use of surgery.

At the present time, many clinicians feel that surgery should be undertaken under primarily two circumstances. The first is shortly after (within approximately four to six weeks) an acute situation in which the disc has suddenly moved out of place and the patient experiences a *closed lock*. When this occurs, most surgeons still recommend between two and six weeks of conservative orthotic therapy first, to see if the disc can be manipulated back into place without surgery. If this fails, surgery is often required.

The second circumstance for surgery occurs when a patient has had continual pain directly from the temporomandibular joint despite all efforts at correction. It is very important, however, that a proper diagnosis be made so that all other possible causes, other than the temporomandibular joint, have been ruled out. It is extremely discouraging for a patient to go through surgery on the temporomandibular joint and have the pain return afterward, due to the fact that the initial cause of pain was not in the joint at all. Fortunately, most surgeons are extremely cautious in this regard.

Even with proper diagnosis, surgery is not a panacea. Occasionally, a patient will still have significant pain even though a good diagnosis was made and excellent surgery performed. Fortunately, this is infrequent.

There are a number of different surgical procedures that can be utilized to help patients with TM dysfunction problems. Surgery may be performed on the jaw joint itself to correct a malfunction or on the jaws in order to correct their positioning, thereby reducing stress on the joint and teeth. The simplest form of surgery, which has developed rather recently, is arthroscopic surgery. This is the same type of surgery, utilizing fiber-optics and very small incisions, which has been performed on patients with knee problems for years. This same procedure can be applied to the temporomandibular joint. It allows the surgeon to limit his surgery to a very small opening, while viewing the joint through a fiber-optic instrument called an arthroscope. Unfortunately, the amount of work that can be done with this instrument is, at present, limited only to viewing inside the joint and flushing out debris in order to loosen any sticky spots. Currently, actual joint repair is only in the experimental stage.

Even arthoscopy should be viewed as a somewhat experimental procedure, even though to date the results have been very favorable. It seems that the mere act of flushing out debris from the joint and mechanically disrupting areas where the joint components have stuck together seems to be all that is necessary to achieve pain relief. Unfortunately, there is no evidence that this type of surgery is actually able to cause the disc to move permanently back into a favorable position. Many practicitioners, including the author, now feel that many patients are able to function without the disc in proper position, provided that they are maintained with splint therapy and an adequate home-care program.

Before arthroscopic surgery was developed, the only type of surgery available consisted of going directly into the joint. This is still the best surgery when it is deemed necessary to reposition and tie the disc back into its proper position. Direct joint surgery also is still the best surgery when there is such significant degeneration in the joints that the remnants of the disc need to be removed and a cushion created between the two bones.

When the disc has slipped out of position yet is basically healthy and not damaged, it is possible for a surgeon literally to pull the disc back into place and suture it into position. The procedure is called a *plication* (ply cayshun). Currently, the success rate for this type of surgery is sixty to seventy percent. It is used most often in an acute situation when the disc slips out of position and the patient experiences a closed lock. The success rate is high because the disc, which has recently slipped, is usually in very good condition, even though the joint ligaments are very loose. Under these conditions, it is possible to pull the disc back into place so that it will be a functioning disc. Unfortunately, if the disc has slipped out for a long time, significant degenerative changes will have taken place. Therefore, even if the surgeon pulls the disc back into place, it is usually not functional. Under these circumstances, the disc must be removed and an attempt made to replace it, either with a man-made substance or some type of scar tissue.

Replacement of discs in previous years was made using different types of man-made materials. However, the long-term success rate with that type of surgery has been relatively low. Currently, surgeons create a cushion between the two bones by placing a man-made material between them for a period of time. Afterward, this material is removed and the resulting scar tissue which has formed around it acts as the cushion. It is a bit early to know what the long-term results of this type of surgery may be; but it appears to be good. In many instances, a similar result can be obtained with the judicious use of different types of orthotics, which, if properly used, may be able to move the joint components in a way that promotes healing and the formation of scar tissue between the two bones.

Surgeons can, when extremely severe degeneration has occurred in the joint, literally add bone to the joint by using a piece of bone from a person's rib or hip. In addition, surgeons can create a mechanical joint using metallic implants. However, these are extreme types of surgery and should be used only in those special cases which can be corrected in no other way. As with all surgery, if there is a conservative way that the patient can be treated, this should be attempted first. Surgery should be resorted to only after all other procedures have failed.

It is extremely important after surgery to correct the surfaces of the teeth and the alignment of the jaw in order to eliminate any destructive forces which may have created the joint problem in the first place. Some of the surgical failures that I have seen are due to the patient's lack of follow-through in having the biting surfaces properly realigned and restored.

ANOTHER TYPE OF SURGERY
Very often, patients will arrive in my office concerned about the possibility of surgery because they knew of someone who had

surgery because of headaches. Since I practice in a medium-sized town, it is not unusual for the patient they are discussing to be one of mine. Often, I find that there is a misunderstanding regarding surgery. People have heard (rightly so) that surgery on the joints should be avoided. They do not know that there is another kind of surgery that is occasionally used to rehabilitate patients with structural problems relating to TM dysfunction. This other type of surgery is not done on the joints themselves; it is done to realign the jaw bones when they are so far out of position that moving them is the only way to align the patient's bite.

As we discussed in Chapter 3, the jaws can grow so poorly that an extremely large pivot is created in the back molar area of the mouth. When this occurs, even drastically reducing the height of the teeth may not be enough to allow the front teeth to touch when the mouth is closed. Under these circumstances, surgery may be necessary in order to realign the bony parts. Often, this surgery removes a section of bone above the back teeth. This tips the upper jaw downward and allows the front teeth to touch again. When the jaw is tipped in this manner, the lower jaw is able to hinge forward providing an added benefit: an improvement in the profile.

To prepare the patient for this type of surgery, it is necessary to place orthodontic appliances. Doing so aligns the teeth and removes any dental compensations. This is done because, during the time the patient's teeth have been out of position, they have moved around in order to accommodate the poor bite. Orthodontics is necessary in order to line up these teeth ideally over their respective jaw bones.

Patients with lower jaw bones that have not grown sufficiently often experience a great deal of muscle spasm in two muscles: the anterior temporalis and the lateral pterygoid. These muscles become severely irritated because patients must constantly project their lower jaws forward while speaking and chewing in order to compensate for their jaw's shortened length. As you can imagine, under these circumstances these muscles will become tired and easily go into spasm.

When the lower jaw has not grown sufficiently forward another type of surgery is needed. Such surgery lengthens the lower jaw, or mandible, and brings it into proper relationship with the upper jaw. As always, a period of orthotic splint therapy is necessary to relieve muscles spasm before the surgery is undertaken.

Occasionally, the lower jaw will grow too large for the upper jaw, or the upper jaw will be too small for the lower jaw. Under such conditions, surgery would move the upper jaw forward or the lower jaw backward, depending on which one is at fault. Sometimes, the upper jaw can be so small that a piece of bone must be inserted to make it larger. (This bone is often taken from the side of the hip.) The results of such surgery can be excellent due to the more relaxed, stable muscle condition that occurs when the muscles are no longer strained because of such poor jaw proportions.

I wish to emphasize that surgery on the joint itself is usually avoided if at all possible. However, realignment of the jaw bones is often useful in order to create proper alignment within the supporting structures, thereby allowing the teeth to be realigned in ideal relationships. As was previously discussed, it is important that orthodontic appliances be utilized to align the teeth before and after the surgical procedure. In addition, the appliances are usually left on during the surgery in order to provide a means by which the surgeon can fix the jaws in position until healing occurs.

If surgery has been recommended, it is important to discuss all possible options with the surgeon prior to making the choice. Fortunately, with jaw realignment surgery, most results are excellent and the complications are few.

REHABILITATING THE MUSCLES: KEEPING THE KINKS OUT
Even though therapy has been successful and the patient is free of pain, it is important not to neglect the muscles. It is important for

muscles which have been subject to trigger points and chronic spasm to be maintained at their maximum length and vitality by a program of stretching and exercise. It is vitally important for you to maintain an awareness of daily activities that may tend to overload the muscles. In addition, stretching exercises learned during the treatment period should be maintained on an ongoing basis to assure that muscles maintain their maximum length. For as a muscle shortens, it becomes more prone to the development of trigger points and the creation of a new pain cycle. Also, a program of regular aerobic exercise can be extremely beneficial for keeping the circulation system and the muscles in a healthier state. By exercising, waste products are removed from your muscles, the metabolism of the muscle is increased, and the utilization of food substances by the muscle tissue is enhanced. All of these factors make the muscles less prone to trigger points and spasm.

In addition, the role of nutrition cannot be diminished after treatment has been successful. A long-term commitment to a healthy eating style can go a long way toward maintaining the proper chemistry for normal pain-free muscle function. Finally, your continued awareness of your daily stress level can be very helpful in heading off potential muscle overload before it occurs. Maintaining a regular program of relaxation techniques, along with strategies such as time management and goal setting, can go a long way toward reducing stress and providing the framework for happy, pain-free living.

CONCLUSION

Relief of pain from TM dysfunction often can be accomplished within a short period of time. However, as you have seen in this chapter, it is extremely important to eliminate the causative factors in order for you to obtain truly lasting, long-term relief. In order to do this, proper placement of the teeth and jaws so that they no longer traumatize your joints or muscles is extremely important, as is maintaining proper chemistry and flexibility in the surrounding muscles. Modifications in lifestyle are the final key to rehabilitation.

In the next chapter, we will talk about your body chemistry and nutrition and how they can have a significant effect on the health of your muscles and the integrity of the TM joint itself.

CHAPTER 9

Vitamins, Minerals & Food: How Vitamin C, B12 and Others Can Help Headaches

I remember when Paul first came to my office; he was an attractive, well-dressed young executive who had a peculiar nervousness about him. He complained of continuous headaches which varied from a dull ache to pain so severe that he described it as a tight metal band crushing his head. At those times, the pain was so intense he could barely function at work. He would not eat supper but would go straight to bed. The following morning, the pain would have subsided to its normal dull ache. Paul said that the headaches usually would begin to intensify around ten o'clock in the morning and would often increase throughout the day, although the pattern was not always the same.

Paul always remembered having headaches rather frequently but had not experienced pain of this severity and duration until the last year when he moved into his new executive position. At first, he thought the pain was due to stress. This diagnosis was confirmed by his family physician. Paul was told to relax and was given muscle relaxants. Bio-feedback therapy was suggested. He took the muscle relaxants which gave him some relief. However, he felt that they interfered with his ability to think clearly at work. So gradually he discontinued them. Besides, he said, "I don't want to take drugs the rest of my life."

Paul went for bio-feedback training which helped to reduce the pain. Unfortunately, he found that he constantly had to be concerned about relaxing his muscles to have any significant effect. Again, this interfered with his ability to function effectively at work and only gave him partial relief. After a while, he used his relaxation techniques less and less, and the headaches continued.

During my examination of Paul, a number of significant factors became apparent. Paul had a bite problem which many people could have tolerated fairly well, However, because of Paul's high stress level and tendency toward clenching, the effects of his bad bite were magnified many times. This contributed to a significant muscle spasm, both in his facial and neck muscles. Even more important, however, was the fact that Paul's diet was horrible. He would arrive at work without eating, usually consuming as much as five or six cups of coffee during the morning. On some days, he would consume a couple of sweet rolls if someone had been kind enough to bring them into the office. Lunch was a "hit or miss affair" depending on the intensity of his schedule. During the afternoon, soda was substituted for coffee. Consumption of five or six cans was not uncommon. Often the only substantial food Paul had during the day was the evening meal. To top all this off, Paul smoked between one and two packs of cigarettes per day.

After a complete examination, I recommended that Paul wear an orthotic splint, undergo physical therapy, and make some major changes in his lifestyle. During the time that it took to have the custom orthotic made, he was able to achieve significant relief on his own. Paul cut back on smoking and enrolled in a stop-smoking program. He began eating a nutritious breakfast and lunch, while cutting the sweets out of his diet and eliminating the caffeine. By the time the orthotic was ready to be placed, his headaches had decreased by almost one-half. Within a month after placing the orthotic and working with his physical therapy, Paul's headaches were gone.

Leann came to my office after hearing me speak at a local function. She had been having headaches for over two years. Although her headaches only occurred a couple of times a week, they were significant enough to keep her from enjoying life to its fullest. She was concerned that there might be a problem with her jaw joints. X-rays of the jaw joints were normal, and Leann's bite was very good. In addition, her jaw muscles were fairly relaxed. However, there were a number of tender spots (trigger points) in her neck muscles. It also became apparent that the onset of her headaches coincided with her beginning to take birth control pills. Since there were no significant factors in her lifestyle which would tend to aggravate the neck muscles, I recommended that she contact her physician about stopping the birth control pills for a few months in order to see what effect they might be having on the headaches. As soon as the birth control pills were stopped, Leann's headaches disappeared. They have not returned.

F ortunately, the human body is a wonderfully resilient mechanism. The abuse we can heap upon it without impairing its normal functioning, is sometimes amazing. Nevertheless, our bodies do have limits and those limits are different for each person. Depending on each person's biologic tolerance level, both structure and stress can overload and thereby create dysfunction and pain in the body's muscle systems.

For muscles to function properly, the chemistry around them must be appropriate. If nutrients are missing, mineral levels are out of line, or hormones are imbalanced, stress and more probably dysfunction, will result in the muscle system. Trigger points can develop or be aggravated after which a "domino effect" can occur, whereby one irritated muscle creates more irritated muscles around it.

Both Paul and Leann suffered from the effects of chemical imbalances, either due to hormonal, nutritional factors, or chemical disruptors. In this chapter, we will be discussing a number of the nutritional and chemical influences on muscle dysfunction. In addition, we will explore ways that nutritionally we may be able to protect yourself against arthritic changes, specifically in the jaw joints and possibly in the rest of your body as well.

HEADACHES COMING AND GOING: CAFFEINE

In our culture, caffeine is widely used as a stimulant. Not only do coffee and tea contain high levels of caffeine (over one hundred milligrams), but caffeine has also been added to many soft drinks because of its mood-elevating effects. In addition, chocolate also contains a significant amount of caffeine.

Caffeine has been linked to a number of metabolic problems. One of the most significant has been cystic breast disease in women. Coffee drinking in excess of three cups per day has been implicated in almost a five-fold increase in pancreatic cancer! It appears that as time goes on more undesirable effects of caffeine will be discovered.

For the person with headaches. we know that caffeine can cause problems in two ways. First, its stimulating affect causes hyper-irritability of muscle tissue. This is just the opposite of what is needed when muscles are already irritated and creating pain. The mechanism for this may be the overall stimulation of the muscles in general. On the other hand, caffeine may specifically stimulate trigger points within the muscles. Second, when a person has consumed a significant amount of caffeine, the blood vessels of the brain will narrow slightly causing reduced blood flow. This, in and of itself, does not necessarily cause headaches. But the discontinuance of caffeine consumption can cause what is called a *rebound headache*, in which the blood vessels, because of a lack of caffeine, overexpand and deliver too much blood to the patient, thus creating a throbbing, pounding headache.

Because of its stimulating effect and a tendency to avoid rebound headaches, patients literally become addicted. For that reason, I usually advise patients to gradually reduce their caffeine intake through means such as substituting decaffeinated coffee for every other cup of regular coffee. A decaffeinated soft drink or fruit juice can also be substituted until the chemical has been eliminated from the diet.

ONE PROBLEM AMONG MANY: TOBACCO

All forms of tobacco contain nicotine; but this is only one compound among many which destroy the health and well-being of tobacco users. However, for the person with headaches, nicotine creates a specific problem. Like caffeine, nicotine is also a muscle irritant. It can aggravate already irritable muscles, creating more pain and spasm. It also may affect trigger points, making them more irritable.

Paradoxically, nicotine also is a *stimulus blocker*. It has a mild sedative effect on the human brain. This is one reason why cigarette smoking tends to be so addictive. People who quit often notice that for the first few days that the world is not as nice a place to live. Noises seem louder and events in general seem harsher. The loss of the nicotine sedative effect creates this phenomenon. (It is interesting to note that nicotine sedates your brain and irritates your muscles simultaneously.) Because many other toxic products are released during tobacco smoking, there is a high possibility that headaches caused by allergic reaction to the compounds released or by a lack of oxygen will result.

SUGAR BLUES: CARBOHYDRATES

One of the great tragedies of our time is the misconception that the most damaging thing about sugar consumption is tooth decay. In reality, probably the least harmful thing that can happen to you when you consume large amounts of simple sugars is that your teeth may become rotten. The damage that occurs within your body chemistry could be far greater.

Our body chemistry has evolved over millions of years. As little as ten thousand years ago, our ancestors ate diets which were high in protein, low in fat, full of complex sugars which released the energies slowly into the system. Body chemistry takes thousands upon thousands of years to change. Therefore, we twentieth century primates are bio-chemically designed for optimum health based on these ancient diets.

Excessive consumption of refined sugar greatly distorts our body chemistry. When sugar enters our blood stream, cells within the pancreas sense the level of sugar present and produce insulin in response to it. Insulin, in turn, is used to metabolize the sugar, transporting it into the individual cells for energy production or transformation into storage as fat molecules.

The ancient design of this system called for the sugars from naturally occurring plants to gradually be released. As these sugars were released, an equivalent amount of insulin was also to be released, thus producing an even release of energy. When refined sugar is ingested it almost immediately produces a large increase in blood sugar, stimulating a huge out-pouring of insulin. This insulin rapidly metabolizes the sugar, converting much of it into fat molecules for storage. This raises triglyceride levels in the blood stream which have been implicated in heart disease.

The story does not end here. Soon, the excess sugar is used up but the insulin is not. This leaves a residual amount of insulin still roaming our circulatory system. This insulin continues to metabolize the remaining sugar in the blood stream, thus dropping the level of sugar (the glucose blood level) below its ideal level for normal body functioning. This condition is called *hypoglycemia* (low blood sugar).

Since a normal level of blood sugar is important for brain function, which requires high amounts of energy, low blood sugar can induce a mild state of depression. This has been referred to as *sugar bl*·· This drop in blood sugar will also trigger headache example of this is the headache which occurs at ten o'clock in the morning in those people who akfast. Because such people have not consumed a of carbohydrates, by mid-morning their sugar level has dropped sufficiently enough to trigger a headache. The sever of such headaches is often increased by the contraction of already overloaded muscles. This occurs because muscles become increasingly irritable at low blood sugar levels. It must be emphasized that ordinary table sugar is not the only sugar responsible for these large variations in blood sugar. Any carbohydrate which tends to release its sugars rapidly into the blood stream can create this type of problem. Natural fruits, which are high in sugar, have this ability and, therefore, should be eaten in moderation. To make matters worse, because of variations in body chemistry, certain individuals are more sensitive or highly reactive to sugars and will tend to produce these swings more easily. Although it is not a cure all, reduction in the consumption of simple sugars along with attention to regular eating habits can go a long way toward reducing the tendency toward head and neck pain.

When blood sugar drops below normal, the natural protective mechanism in your body creates a craving for more sugar, thus beginning a vicious cycle. This is why sugar and other simple carbohydrates tend to be mildly addicting. (It is interesting to note that food manufacturers also are aware of this. If you read labels carefully, you will find sugar in a great many prepared food products which should require absolutely no sugar at all for good taste. The mild addictive nature of sugar automatically increases the demand for their product.)

VITAMINS
Our body is composed of trillions of cells, each containing billions of even smaller chemical factories. The chemical reactions occurring in these factories require helpers, known as catalysts, in order to be able to combine, disconnect, and rearrange the various molecules necessary to maintain and support the human body. Many of these catalysts are vitamins, most of which are unavailable except from sources outside of our bodies. There are many fine publications which deal with the individual vitamins, the diseases

...ı deficiency, and optimum vitamin levels. How-
...only with those that have a specific relation with
...scles and the possible production of headaches.

Folic Acid. Folic acid is required for a number of important chemical reactions within the muscle structure, in addition to being important for normal brain function. Individuals who are deficient in folic acid will often experience muscles which are irritable and very susceptible to trigger point spasms. For these individuals, headache pain is frequent. They may also suffer from the additional symptoms of diarrhea, a sore tongue, and dizziness when arising from a sitting or lying down position (orthostatic hypotension). Depending on the severity of the problem, such people also may experience anemia, clotting problems, weight loss, fever, and problems of malabsorption.

Because folic acid is not stored in the body, deficiencies can be related to an insufficient amount in the diet or problems with intestinal absorption. Please remember that each individual is different bio-chemically. Therefore, people's ability to absorb any vitamin is going to vary greatly. (That is why the F.D.A. minimum daily requirement for vitamins is similar to trying to provide everyone in the country with the same size shoes.) Another cause of folic acid deficiency can be excessive and hard use of muscles, which burn the folic acid out of the system. Injury or surgery also will use excessive amounts of folic acid. Severe emotional stress also burns up great amounts of folic acid. It is not unusual to find people under severe emotional stress that suffer from headache problems and trigger points. The connection here should not be overlooked.

Hyperactivity of the glandular system may create a condition known as hypermetabolism (hyperthyroidism). In this condition, the body chemistry functions at an accelerated rate. This problem may require the addition of large amounts of folic acid into the system in order to avoid a state of deficiency. In addition, the following conditions may also precipitate a deficiency of folic acid: severe illnesses, severe liver disease, severe infections, and disorders of the gastrointestinal tract.

Alcohol tends to burn a number of vitamins out of the body, creating deficiency states when consumed in high concentrations. However, even moderate consumption can reduce tissue levels of certain vitamins, especially folic acid, which are required for optimum muscle function. Also, certain medications react with folic acid, removing it from the body. For instance, many anti-inflammatory medications remove folic acid from the body. Naprosyn, Motrin, Nuprin, Aspirin and Advil are only a few. It is not uncommon for patients who experience significant head and neck pain to have taken these anti-inflammatory drugs over a long period of time. Unfortunately, in doing so they may be perpetuating their problem by reducing folic acid and, therefore, increasing muscle irritability simultaneously. Anti-convulsants, such as Dilantin, also remove folic acid. So do oral contraceptives. In addition, anti-tubercular drugs, along with special folic acid antagonists used in the treatment of a malignancy, will also reduce folic acid levels.

Without sufficient intake, it takes approximately five months to deplete the body of its folic acid reserves. This time period can be reduced, however, if the person is subject to severe trauma, kidney failure, or extensive surgical procedures.

The dietary sources of folic acid are leafy vegetables, yeast, liver and other organ meats. Fresh uncooked fruit, fresh fruit juice, lightly cooked fresh, green vegetables such as broccoli or asparagus are also sources of folic acid. (Please note: folic acid is easily destroyed by cooking and processing foods.)

Vitamin B-12. A severe deficiency of vitamin B-12, or cobalamin as it is medically termed, will cause pernicious anemia and eventually death. One of the more common symptoms of low B-12 levels is increased susceptibility of the muscles to trigger point spasms. In addition, several other symptoms are common: constipation, headache, agitation, mood changes, fatigue, depression, burning, numbness. Tingling in the hands or feet and orthostatic hypotension, which is feeling faint or dizzy upon arising rapidly, are also symptoms. Vitamin B-12 deficiency causes these varied symptoms because it is an element in numerous chemical reactions within the body, such as protein synthesis and fat and carbohydrate metabolism.

Since B-12 is not stored within the body, one significant cause of B-12 deficiency is insufficient dietary intake. However, individual body abnormalities may cause a lack of adequate absorption, although a person may be consuming an adequate quantity of the vitamin. Other causes of B-12 deficiency are severe emotional stress, significant injuries or surgery, and hypermetabolism. As with folic acid, liver disease, severe illness, infections, or genetic problems of utilization also contribute to vitamin B-12 deficiencies. One interesting way that B-12 is depleted from the body is through excessive and hard use of our muscles. This may be one reason why patients who have inadequate dietary uptake or absorption, develop trigger points so easily when even moderate exercise is performed.

B-12 is unique because it is found principally in bacteria. It is not found in plants unless they are contaminated by bacteria. The richest food sources of vitamin B-12 are liver, kidney, shell fish, fish, poultry, egg yolk, and fermented cheeses.

Vitamin C. Vitamin C is probably the most well-known vitamin. It, however, is often one of the most misunderstood. A lack of vitamin C produces a disease called *scurvy*. Scurvy prevents the body from manufacturing sufficient collagen. (Collagen constitutes nearly one-quarter of the protein in body tissues. It is the primary component in ligaments, tendons, and the walls of our blood vessels. Without it, we are more prone to injury and bruising.) When people have scurvy they suffer from weakness, lassitude, irritability, and aching pain. In addition, their gums become swollen and bleed easily. Often their teeth become loose and fall out. If untreated, scurvy eventually will lead to death.

In addition to the production of collagen, vitamin C is essential for the synthesis of two brain chemicals: epinephrine and sero-tonin. Vitamin C also protects the enzymes which aid in keeping toxic substances from damaging our body chemistry. Vitamin C also is an important building block for stress hormones released by our adrenal glands.

Unfortunately, vitamin C is not synthesized by the body; there-fore, it is not stored by the body. Consequently, for people to maintain adequate tissue health, sufficient daily intake is required. At this time in the United States, the basic recommended daily allowance for vitamin C is between sixty and eighty milligrams per day. For many individuals this may be considerably below the level necessary to maintain optimum health. (An interesting note: It is estimated that our pre-historic ancestors consumed approximately 600mg of vitamin C daily, due to their all natural fresh diet.)

Factors such as smoking, which greatly increases the loss of vitamin C in the liver; alcohol, which burns vitamin C from the body; stress, which depletes vitamin C by utilizing it in the production of adrenal hormones; and basic variations in our body's ability to absorb and utilize vitamin C make the minimum daily requirement inaccurate. Additionally, women who take birth control pills may discover they need a vitamin C increase by three to ten fold.

In our office, we use a quick test called the lingual ascorbic acid test, which provides an approximation of a person's vitamin C level. In addition, blood tests that determine vitamin C levels in the blood stream are available. In order to maintain adequate levels of vitamin C within the body, many people take between 500 and 1000 milligrams per day. However, this amount will vary greatly, depending on each individual's lifestyle and stress factors.

Vitamin B-1 (Thiamine). A severe lack of thiamine causes the disease called *beri-beri*, a neurological disease that, if left untreated, can result in death. The first known treatment for this disease occurred in 1884 when meat, vegetables, and condensed milk were added to the rice diet of Japanese sailors, reducing death by beri-beri. By 1936, the structure and synthesis of this vitamin had been accomplished. Vitamin B-1 functions by forming a critical link in the production of energy within the muscles. In addition, vitamin B-1 is central in the formation of two amino acids necessary for brain function.

The symptoms of thiamine deficiency are very similar to those of B-12 deficiency. Such symptoms include: mood changes, depression, agitation, insomnia, generalized weakness, and blood pressure changes. Of significant importance to people suffering from head and neck pain is the fact that thiamine deficiency increases a person's susceptibility to trigger points in the muscles. This last fact can make people more resistant to physical therapy or treatment because their muscles are in, and will remain in, an untreatable condition.

Borderline thiamine deficiency tends to be fairly common in the general population and is not always related to a lack of adequate intake. In many individuals, there seems to be a problem with intestinal absorption and, even though large amounts of thiamine are given orally, adequate blood levels are not obtained. Therefore, even though you may be eating well and are taking vitamins, you still may have a low vitamin B-1 level. This is easily determined with a blood test. If the blood level is low, even after taking vitamin B-1 orally, injections may be necessary to correct the problem.

An insufficiency or deficiency of thiamine may be due to insufficient intake, excessive alcohol ingestion, liver injury, magnesium deficiency, or antacids. In addition, the tannin in tea will bind with this vitamin making it unavailable for absorption into the body. Diuretics used for water retention also will purge this vitamin from the body. The regular consumption of large amounts of water may also wash the vitamin away. Those people with liver disease will have a problem with transforming the vitamin into a form that can be used by the body.

High consumption of sugar, in certain individuals, may use up available thiamine supplies, especially if they are marginal. This also will create a thiamine deficiency. (The author feels high consumption of sugar may be one reason why some people who have extremely poor diets suffer from muscle spasm that does not respond easily to routine treatment programs.)

I would like to repeat again: It is important to remember that the levels of these important vitamins within the body should not be taken for granted. Variations in the ability of a person's body to absorb a vitamin and utilize it, along with significant variations in diet, can produce borderline states of deficiency which contribute to needless aggravation of head and neck pain.

Sources of thiamine are pork, beans, nuts, certain whole grain cereals, kidney, liver, and beef. Eggs and fish also contain helpful amounts. (Remember: vitamin B-1 is quickly destroyed above 212 degrees Fahrenheit (boiling) and is leached out of foods by washing.)

DIETARY MINERALS AND TRACE ELEMENTS

In order to maintain optimal functioning of muscle tissue, several minerals are especially important. They are calcium, potassium, iron, and magnesium.

Calcium. Calcium is essential for normal muscle contraction. The importance of calcium in normal membrane function is also now being recognized. The daily recommended allowance of calcium is 800 milligrams per day. However, 1000 milligrams per day or more may be necessary to maintain adequate levels in middle-aged or elderly individuals. Two servings daily from the milk group will provide adequate levels of calcium for most individuals. However, the protein in cow's milk has been implicated in a number of both severe and mild allergic reactions. Fortunately, a few other foods besides milk contain calcium. Some are: green leafy vegetables, legumes, canned salmon, oysters, clams, dried fruits, and soy bean curd. If a person cannot tolerate dietary sources, a supplement such as calcium phosphate or calcium carbonate can be taken. As we become older, the level of hydrochloric acid in our stomachs tends to decrease, reducing the absorption of calcium. To overcome this, calcium citrate can be taken.

Potassium. Potassium also is needed for normal muscle contraction. A diet high in fat, refined sugar and over-salted food, which is low in potassium, can lead to a potassium deficiency. In addition, laxatives, certain diuretics, and diarrhea can increase potassium loss. The recommended daily allowance for potassium is approximately two grams. Good sources of potassium are fruits, especially bananas and citrus fruits, potatoes, green leafy vegetables, wheat germ, beans, lentils, prunes, nuts, and dates. (Note: Levels within the normal range, but in the lower third, can create in some individuals significant irritability in the muscles.)

Iron. People who have low iron levels are called anemic. In this condition, oxygen transport within the blood stream is limited. This impairs energy production in the muscles. One of the most common causes of iron deficiency is excessive loss of blood, without adequate dietary replacement of the iron lost. Women are especially prone to this problem because of their monthly cycle. The recommended daily allowance of iron is 1.8 milligrams. Liver, meats, organ meats, deep green leafy vegetables, peas, beans, whole grain cereals and bread, dried fruits, shellfish, and egg yolks are all rich in iron.

Magnesium. Magnesium plays an essential role in the ability of individual muscle fibers to contract. Magnesium also plays an a key role in many essential enzymatic reactions. The recommended daily allowance for magnesium is 350 milligrams per day for adult men and 300 milligrams per day for adult women. Many good calcium supplements also contain the minimum daily requirement of magnesium. This type of supplement is highly recommended. It is important to note that magnesium toxicity can occur in elderly people who constantly take antacids or laxatives containing magnesium. It is important to be aware of this possibility and take precautions against it.

VITAMIN C AND KEEPING THE JOINTS SLIPPERY

The joints in our body are magnificently engineered. The friction within a human joint is ten times less than the most sophisticated ball bearing man can make. The friction within a human joint is about the same as the friction generated by a hockey puck sliding on ice. Yet, any surgeon who has operated on the temporomandibular joint will tell you that often times the lubricant in the joint has become thick and the joint surfaces have become sticky, forming what are called *adhesions*. Adhesions are fibrous connections binding down and reducing the movement within the joint. Often, the surgeon will go into the joint with an instrument called an arthroscope and flush out the joint while gently removing the adhesions. This action helps the joint regain its motion and flexibility.

These sticky joints may develop because of the overloading and trauma a joint receives due to bad bites, excessive bruxing, and clenching. Such trauma and overloading leads to inflammation. Unfortunately, in the presence of inflammation the joint lubricant called *hyaluronic acid* is rapidly destroyed by an enzyme called *hyaluronidase*. As a result, the joint begins to lose its lubrication and friction increases. This leads to increased inflammation, and the process becomes a vicious cycle. Even with the skilled work of a surgeon who can remove damage within the joint, flushing out debris and restoring mobility, the potential for recurrence is high. Although, reducing pressures within the joint space, through orthotics and improvement of the bite, may help, vitamin C may also play an extremely important role in helping to break this vicious cycle.

Under high concentrations of vitamin C, hyaluronidase, the enzyme which breaks down the lubrication within the joint spaces, is inhibited. Thus, the hyaluronic acid (or joint lubricant) is maintained at its optimum levels, thereby reducing friction. This protective action of vitamin C may not be limited to the temporo-mandibular joints. This therapeutic affect could be a significant factor in helping to reduce long-term degenerative changes (arthritis) in other joints of your body. (Remember, however, that there are many other factors involved in arthritic degeneration beside trauma and reduction of joint lubrication. However, significantly reducing trauma and maintaining vitamin C levels may help many individuals.) Because body chemistries vary greatly, a daily intake of one gram or more of vitamin C may be necessary to provide this effect.

VITAMIN E: THE PAIN RELIEVER

Eighteen years ago, when I graduated from dental school, vitamin E was literally on the back shelf and considered of little practical value. Over the years, a great deal has been learned about this important vitamin, which functions in many different ways. One of the most important effects of vitamin E seems to be its ability to perform the duties of an *anti-oxidant*.

Through normal metabolism and also due to injury, compounds called *free radicals* are released . (When I as younger, free radicals were considered those who had been let out of jail.) However, in this instance, we are talking about a chemical that has the ability to aggressively latch on to another chemical and, thereby damage it. If this chemical happens to be DNA or RNA, the chemical building blocks of the body, significant damage could result. Some people believe one of the mechanisms for cancer development is damage to our genetic DNA molecules due to free radical attack.

A classic example of free radical damage is radiation poisoning.

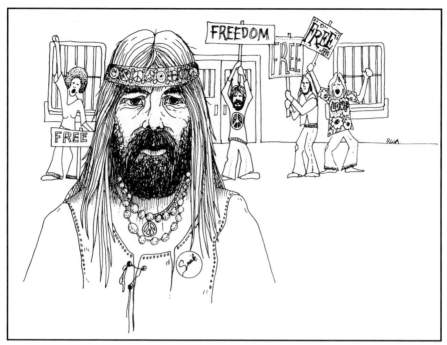

Free Radicals

Ionizing radiation, when passing through the body, changes the chemical composition of many of the compounds in our body, turning them into free radicals. These, in turn, attack other chemicals. When enough free radicals are produced, radiation sickness develops.

When considering damage to the temporomandibular joints, you must recognize that during normal, everyday metabolism, free radicals are generated by the cells in and around the body's joints. As we have learned, structural problems and waste product pile up can lead to a higher concentration of these free radicals in certain areas of the joint, possibly creating damage. In addition, when a joint is injured, even slightly, red blood cells may be pushed into the joint space where they become ruptured, releasing copper and iron ions which also act as free radicals. The more free radicals that are produced, the more damage is done. The more damage done, the more free radicals are produced. Thus, a vicious cycle ensues.

Vitamin E, because it is an anti-oxidant, has the ability to grab on to these free radicals and remove them from circulation before they can damage surrounding tissues. Although this occurs in all areas of the body, it is especially important in our joints.

The effectiveness of vitamin E as a pain reliever has been demonstrated by a carefully controlled study in Germany. This study compared vitamin E to a popular medication commonly used for arthritis pain relief. When a dose of 400 International Units of vitamin E was given daily, those patients suffering from osteoarthritis received the same pain relief as those receiving the more popular medication. How the vitamin E brought about the pain relief was unclear. However, the elimination of free radicals may have been the chief mechanism involved.

Although vitamin E is one of the fat soluble vitamins, it is not stored adequately within the body and is only adequately available in very fresh, recently picked fruits and vegetables. Unfortunately, because of storage and transportation, the vitamin E level in the foods we eat deteriorates rapidly. Again, a dosage level of approximately 400 International Units seems to be effective for arthritis. (NOTE: Taking over 600 International Units of vitamin E daily may result in harmful side effects.)

SELENIUM

In addition to vitamin C and vitamin E, both selenium and betacarotene may be useful in reducing the potential for arthritic degeneration, especially within the temporomandibular joints. Selenium is an important trace mineral that has significant anti-oxidant properties. Unfortunately, selenium is not stored in our bodies, and its availability in our diets has been significantly reduced because it is easily depleted from the soil. Years of continuous farming have generally reduced selenium in plant products to an almost negligible amount. Because of this, the chances of us gaining adequate selenium through normal dietary intake are slim. Supplementation of up to 200 micrograms a day seems to be useful. In the case of selenium, a little bit may be good, however, a lot will definitely not be better. Selenium is toxic in high levels and, therefore, should not be taken in excess.

BETACAROTENE

Betacarotene, a compound which turns into vitamin A within the body, is abundant in green leafy vegetables such as broccoli and Brussels sprouts. Betacarotene is only turned into vitamin A when there is a demand for it by the body. Therefore, the tendency toward toxicity is greatly reduced. However, in some individuals there seems to be a tendency to convert betacarotene into vitamin A more readily, thus providing the possibility for some toxicity to occur. Because of this, it would be wise to limit supplementation of this vitamin to no more than 15 milligrams per day, preferably under the supervision of a professional.

The anti-oxidant effect of betacarotene may be very helpful in reducing the potential for damage within the joint spaces. In addition, betacarotene has the ability to make significant improvements in pre-cancerous cells by helping them change back to a more normal state. A significant amount of research has been done in this regard. A Canadian study found that those patients who had high intake of green leafy vegetables containing betacarotene, even though they were smokers, had cancer rates almost the same as non-smokers. The study also found that those patients who had very low intakes of betacarotene and smoked ended up with high rates of lung cancer. In the future, betacarotene and its derivatives may play an important role in the prevention and treatment of a number of ailments and in our overall, better health.

CONCLUSION

Because our bodies are so adaptable, and because bio-chemical changes within our bodies tend to be subtle and take place over time, it is very easy to minimize the effects that proper nutrition and vitamin supplementation may have on our health and well-being.

In addition, the biochemical individuality of each person creates a situation in which some nutrients may be absorbed and utilized very well while other nutrients are not, thus setting the stage for sub-clinical deficiency.

In this chapter, we have seen how your muscles and temporomandibular joints may be adversely affected or enhanced, depending on the levels of several vitamins and minerals. In addition, a diet which is low in red meat and higher in fish and vegetables can provide you with a physiological environment in which inflammation is much less likely to occur. Habits such as smoking and consuming large amounts of caffeine or sugar have been shown to lead to painful muscle spasm and even depression. However, you do have a choice, and you can eat better to feel better now!

CHAPTER 10

Preventing Pain: Protecting Your Joints and Muscles

When she first arrived in our office, Marilyn was suffering from severe headaches which occurred almost every other day. The pain would begin below her eyes, increasing in intensity until, as she described it, "both eyeballs felt as though they were on fire." As the headache continued, the pain would extend around the entire top of her head. The pain was seriously disrupting not only her work, but also her family life. Many nights Marilyn would go directly to bed without even fixing supper or spending time with her family.

Marilyn had first suspected that she might have a sinus problem and visited her physician who then referred her to an ear, nose, and throat specialist. After a thorough evaluation, he could find nothing wrong, although he suspected a mild sinus irritation and prescribed antihistamines. This provided some mild relief. However, Marilyn continued to seek help and was referred to my office by a neurologist who was very suspicious that the problem might be related to her chewing apparatus.

My examination of Marilyn revealed that many of her facial

muscles were extremely tender to touch. In addition, her trapezius muscle, which is the large muscle covering the upper third of the back, also had numerous trigger points. Marilyn related to me that she had had occasional headaches before things really got bad. However, approximately eight months ago she had gone through an extremely stressful period, and that is when the really bad headaches had begun. Even though the stress had passed, the headaches had remained and things even seemed to be getting worse.

The x-rays which we recommended were quite revealing. They showed a significant amount of degeneration in both the left and right temporomandibular joints. We proceeded with orthotic therapy, along with physical therapy to relax the muscles as much as possible. Relief was rapid; within a month, Marilyn was feeling considerably better. Her headaches had decreased to one or two a month and the severity was much less. We continued working with Marilyn and reached a state where her headaches occurred only rarely. When the tenderness had left her muscles and her temporomandibular joints, we evaluated the fit of her teeth and recommended orthodontic treatment to eliminate bumping of the teeth, which aggravated the muscles and most likely contributed to the degeneration of her temporomandibular joints.

We had made Marilyn retainers and things were progressing wonderfully when she returned to my office one day quite upset. She said that she had had a severe headache the day before, and she was extremely concerned that her headaches were returning. We started to talk, and it soon became apparent that Marilyn was no longer doing a number of important things which she had been instructed to continue. For instance, she was not wearing her orthotic at night in order to rest her arthritic joints. She had also begun to neglect her stretching exercises, prescribed to help maintain flexibility and length in her facial and neck muscles. Moreover, when she noticed that she was beginning to feel some discomfort, she neglected to apply moist heat to the sore muscles as quickly as possible. Marilyn and I discussed the fact that we could never make her temporo-mandibular joints brand new, which meant that some effort and maintenance would be required for her to remain pain-free. Marilyn recommitted to taking the proper and necessary actions. She wanted to prevent future headaches for herself and wanted to know how to help her friends and children prevent them also.

M arilyn is not alone in her concern for pre of head and neck pain; many patients v share the same concern. They want to kno.. and neck pain happen and how both can be prevented. These people want to make sure that it does not happen to their children or to their friends and relatives.

Some people are angry with the medical and dental profession for not having prevented the problem. But in all fairness to physicians and dentists, it is important for patients to understand that in years past professionals simply did not know enough to help them with the problem or to prevent the problem from occurring. In fact, most practitioners (unless they were trained within the last five years) received little or no instruction in the diagnosis and treatment of TM dysfunction. Even today, the diagnosis and treatment of this problem is surrounded by a great deal of controversy regarding how to treat it, when to treat it, and in some circles, if the problem even exists at all.

The difficulty with diagnosing TM dysfunction lies in the nature of the disease itself. TM dysfunction is multi-factorial. This simply means that there are many causative factors related to head and neck pain. In addition, TM dysfunction is the great imposter; it mimics many other diseases and, therefore, is easily incorrectly diagnosed.

Physicians, through no fault of their own, have received little or no training in the area of TM dysfunction. Therefore, they may not diagnose the problem properly. Unfortunately, to treat and diagnose TM problems well, both the input of the physician and dentist are extremely important. This is true because TM dysfunction is a medical problem with a dental component.

There is good news, however. Today there are many new methods for preventing head and neck pain problems from occurring or reoccurring. In this chapter, then, we will discuss a number of ways that you can help yourself and your friends avoid the nagging and annoying TM dysfunction problem.

AKE CARE OF YOUR TEETH SO THEY WILL
TAKE CARE OF YOU

I cannot emphasize enough how important it is to maintain a full compliment of teeth which are healthy and in proper alignment. Of course, for years dentists have been telling us that we should brush our teeth and get frequent check-ups so that we can have a beautiful smile and be free of dental pain. However, as our knowledge grows with regard to temporomandibular function and dysfunction, we in the dental profession are finding that maintenance of one's teeth is absolutely essential to maintaining the health and integrity of the jaw joints and chewing muscles.

The reason teeth are so critical to jaw function (and therefore to headache pain) has to do with two things: the mechanical loading of the jaw joint itself and the potential for bumping and banging the teeth together. Let's discuss the damage caused by losing tooth structure or teeth first.

Recent research indicates that the jaw joints are not meant to support the entire load of the forces exerted by chewing. Estimates range from forty to sixty percent of our chewing force is actually transmitted to the joints. In order for the load to be properly distributed, it is absolutely essential that the teeth be there to support the bite. If, through neglect or injury, teeth are damaged so that part of their top portion or crown is lost, or the tooth itself is lost, the support of that tooth will no longer be present. Therefore, that portion of the load will be transferred to the jaw joint. Thus, the more teeth that are lost, the heavier the load placed upon the joints (See Figure 10.1).

When the temporomandibular joints become overloaded, the cartilage and disc within them may begin to undergo changes. The cartilage may develop small cracks or fissures, and, eventually, the underlying bone can become thicker. The disc will also begin to show signs of wear and breakdown. The rate at which these changes occur varies from individual to individual and often is dependent on the structure of the jaw or the amount of clenching

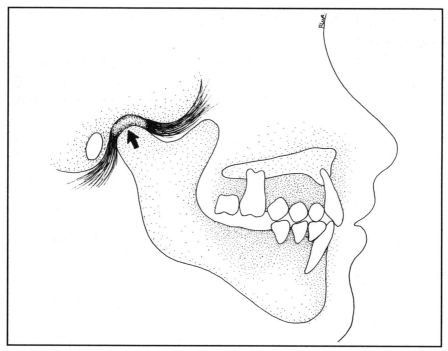

Figure 10.1

and grinding the patient does. For example, a person who has a wide face with a square jaw line already has very strong jaw muscles. In this particular individual, loss of supporting tooth structure will immediately throw heavier loads onto the joints. On the other hand, a person with a long, narrow face may not develop problems quite as rapidly or at all, because of the lighter forces placed on the joints.

A more serious problem occurs when tooth material is lost on only one side of the jaw. In such cases, because of the lack of symmetry, the potential exists for torquing, twisting, or other damaging forces to be generated within the joint on the opposite side, thereby injuring cartilage and ligaments. At the present time, we do not understand completely all the different forces that are generated within the joints. However, after a person loses teeth, we can often see the impact on the temporomandibular joints within a few years. For instance, joints may begin clicking because the disc has been pushed out of position, or the fluid within the disc has become sticky and less lubricating. After a while, significant changes may be evident on an x-ray, such as a wearing down of the head or condyle of the lower jaw. After more time, definite degenerative arthritic changes may be seen on an x-ray.

Maintaining sufficient tooth support is critical to the health of the joints. This can be done by replacing any missing teeth, preferably with something that is stable and not removable such as bridgework or fixed implants, as opposed to partial or full removable dentures. The reason for this is that removable replacements must often rest on the surface of the gum tissue. Unfortunately, pressure directly on the gum tissue causes resorption or shrinkage of the bone underneath, reducing its ability to support the bite and, thereby, transferring the force to the temporomandibular joints. On the other hand, with bridgework, which is supported on either end by a tooth, or with an implant, which is put directly into the bone, there is no shrinkage and proper support of the temporomandibular joints can be maintained.

However, what if you do have a removable partial or a denture? Does this mean that degeneration of the joints is inevitable? Not necessarily. When the person makes sure that the appliances are maintained, that is, adjusted or realigned at regular intervals so that proper support of the joints can be maintained, then the process of degeneration may be significantly reduced or eliminated.

Occasionally, some patients may experience what is termed rapid turnover of bone. For them, changes within the bones that support the partial or denture will occur much more rapidly and, therefore, maintenance must be more frequent. However, there is another important fact to consider if this is the case. Rapid changes in bone shape or bone loss may indicate a more serious problem which could eventually lead to osteoporosis. Therefore, it would be well-advised for anyone experiencing significant bone loss under

their dental appliances or around existing te
osteoporosis evaluation done by their physiciar

Any rapid change or turnover rate in bone may alsu .
affect the health of the temporomandibular joints, as well as othei
joints within the body. Unfortunately, damage to the temporomandibular joints is often not immediately painful. If it were, more
people would seek correction and treatment before any significant
damage had been done. Consequently, many people wait a great
deal of time without rebuilding or replacing their teeth and,
therefore, may greatly compromise the health of their temporomandibular joints for the rest of their lives.

GREAT FITTING TEETH MEAN HEALTHY TEETH
AND HEALTHY JOINTS

One of the principle factors affecting the development of TM
dysfunction is teeth which do not fit properly. This is called
malocclusion (bad bite). Because of the tremendous forces the
chewing muscles exert on the jaw joints, improper positioning of
one or more of the teeth can greatly alter the dynamics of jaw
movements. For example, a tooth which is significantly out of
position will simply not be there to support the bite. On the other
hand, a tooth which is too high will cause the jaw to tip, placing
undesirable torque and load on the joints.

Because our bodies have a magnificent, protective mechanism,
our brain will remember which teeth do not fit properly and will
use that information to protect the teeth while guiding the jaw
closed. Unfortunately, in protecting the teeth, adverse forces may
be transferred to the jaw joints. Moreover, the muscles will become
fatigued and irritable trying to perform the intricate movements
necessary to avoid improperly positioned teeth.

Having poorly fitting teeth is similar to having a stone in your
shoe. That is, you can probably learn to walk with it; but eventually
you will develop a callous under your foot in order to be able to
function more normally. As time goes on, though, you w

experience more and more back pain due to the unusual movements you would need to perform in order to walk. Eventually, you
might also develop arthritis in the spine, and possibly even the knee
and hip joints. The jaw joints, and their supporting musculature, are
no different.

One important aspect of crooked teeth is a problem called a *cross
bite*. It is normal for the upper arch of teeth to slightly overlap the
lower arch. A cross bite occurs when the reverse is true: when an
upper tooth is inside a lower tooth. (See Figure 10.2). This
positioning problem, especially when it occurs in the back teeth,
creates significant overloading of the joints and muscles. I have
seen a cross bite create jaw problems so often, that I felt it needed
special mention here. I should add that cross bites in children
potentially are very damaging to the development of the jaw joints
and should be corrected as soon as possible.

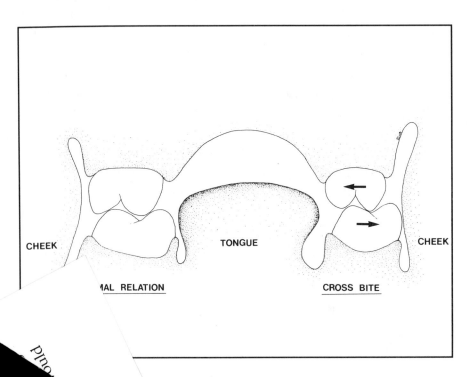

TELL-TALE SIGNS: A HINT OF TROUBLE

One very important sign that there is a problem with the alignment of the teeth is an accelerated wearing-down of the tooth surfaces. If a number of teeth are worn down significantly and you are experiencing head and neck pain, there is a strong probability that one of the contributing causes is tooth or jaw alignment. (Please note here that we are not talking about wearing the teeth down to the bone; we are talking about wear that is significant enough to be noticed. Of course, some wear is normal as we age. However, when teeth are well-aligned, this wear is usually minimal.)

There are a number of things which can increase the wearing down of teeth. The most obvious is excessive clenching and grinding of the teeth. This may be due to stress, or it may be due to the body's inherent desire to rid itself of noxious irritants, such as the point of a tooth which gets in the way of ideal jaw function. In such a case, grinding and clenching may be increased in an attempt to wear away this problem area. However, in the process other teeth also become worn.

Wearing of teeth is also complicated by the fact that some teeth tend to be more dominant. Therefore, in chewing and grinding movements, our body will unconsciously try to avoid these dominant teeth and in doing so will wear down teeth in other parts of the mouth. A classic example of this is a wearing down of the canines or eye teeth. These teeth are found in the front corners of your mouth. They should be slightly pointed and usually will have a heavy or more prominent root. (By rubbing your finger over the roots of your front teeth you may notice this prominence.)

The canines or eye teeth should be pointed. When they are flattened off, it is a sign that one of the big molars on the opposite side of your mouth in the back is bumping. If the molars are out of position, the jaw, because of their dominance, avoids them when closing. In doing so, the eye teeth are worn down.

If pain is present in the above situation, it first should be dealt by means of orthotics, physical therapy, or other non-surgery treatments which have been discussed. Then, the person's bite can be analyzed and the high spots removed. Very often, patients will ask: "Why can't we just grind on the tooth in order to relieve the problem?" This sounds pretty simple and seems to make sense. However, when any pain is present, muscles will be under tension in order to restrict movement of the painful parts. When this occurs, it is impossible to relax the jaws enough so that the "high spot" or bumping tooth can be found. Therefore, if the tooth were ground down without relieving the muscle spasm, there is a very strong probability that either the wrong area would be reshaped or that the reshaping and recontouring would be incomplete. Under these circumstances, the person may not get well at all or they would feel better only for a short time, with the pain gradually returning.

Teeth can also wear excessively when the jaws themselves are significantly out of position. You will remember from Chapter Five that those individuals with wide, square facial patterns and deep overlap of their front teeth show excessive amounts of wear on the lower front teeth and often on the backs of the upper front teeth. On the other hand, those people with very long, narrow faces show large amounts of wear on the back teeth. This wear is an extremely important clue as to where the pressure is being applied to where the overloading is occurring. Again, in these instances, once the pain has been removed the bite can be accurately analyzed and appropriate measures can be taken to realign teeth. And in the most severe instances, steps can be taken to realign the jaw structure.

PROTECT THE MUSCLES, PERFECT THE POSTURE

Since a great deal of the discomfort associated with head and neck pain comes from muscle pain, maintenance of a healthy, flexible muscle structure becomes extremely important. I find it tragic when older individuals come into my office for help with head and neck pain problems and there has been significant degeneration in the neck, often due to poor posture over a lifetime.

A forward head posture, where the head is continually tipped forward on the spine, is one of the most damaging habits you can have. (See Figure 10.3) Forward head postures may be due, in part, to an inherent, structural defect. However, often the problem begins in youth with a slouched shoulder position, which pulls on the neck and causes the head to drop forward. Rather than look at the ground, the most natural act in this position, the people tip their head up slightly in order to look forward. This puts an excessive strain on the muscles in the back of the neck.

Most bowling balls weigh from seven to ten pounds. This is the approximate weight of a human head. Imagine the pressure on the neck muscles when the head is in a forward position. After years in this abnormal position, arthritis may develop in the neck vertebrae, creating a problem which can never be completely corrected. In addition, many years of a forward head position strain the muscles so much that numerous trigger points can develop in the neck and shoulder area. This adds to the discomfort.

If a structural imbalance of the bite is present, the extra stress, which is thrown into the neck area, can easily cause pain. This occurs because the head is balanced on the shoulders and any increase in muscle tension in the front of the head (chewing and muscles in front of the neck) must be counterbalanced by an increase in muscle tension in the back of the head. (The reverse is also true.) Thus, many times dental orthotic splints improve neck problems, because they relieve the strain on the front muscles of the head which, in turn, relieves the strain on the back muscles of the head. In addition, the dental orthotic changes the head's center of gravity and causes the lower jaw to become slightly repositioned. This reduces the load on the muscles at the back of the neck. The longer poor posture has existed, the more difficult the resulting damage is to correct, and the more limited the final result will be.

Therefore, it is extremely important to maintain good posture habits in order to avoid overload of the neck muscles and vertebrae. When standing, maintain a head upright, shoulders back position.

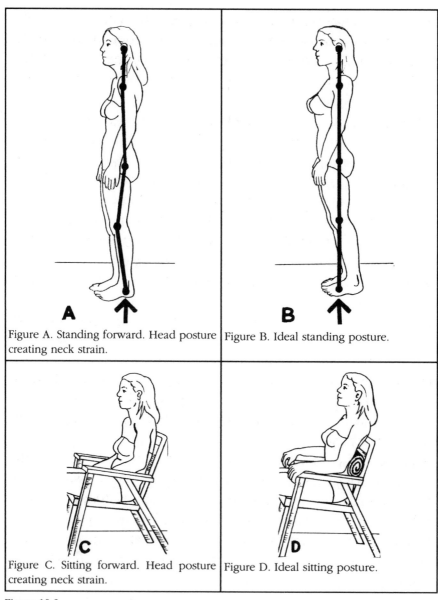

Figure A. Standing forward. Head posture creating neck strain.

Figure B. Ideal standing posture.

Figure C. Sitting forward. Head posture creating neck strain.

Figure D. Ideal sitting posture.

Figure 10.3

Do not allow the shoulders nor the head to drop forward. For some people, this position may be uncomfortable at first. In addition, this position will require some stretching and retraining of muscles using the exercises on the following pages. Occasionally, the help of a physical therapist may be necessary in order to completely relax and mobilize the shortened muscles. Nevertheless, all of this trouble is well worth the added pain and problems you might otherwise encounter.

Throughout the day, it is important to maintain good work and posture habits. Important concepts to remember are: do not allow the head to be in a forward position, and do not allow the muscles to maintain any unusual position for any length of time. Both of these can initiate muscle spasms. For example, don't hold a telephone between your head and your ear. When working at a desk, prop your work materials up so that you are not leaning over your work. If working at a computer terminal, lower your chair or raise the work area so that tipping the head forward when viewing the work is not necessary. If, for some reason, it is necessary to keep the head in an unusual position for any length of time, provide your muscles with frequent breaks by straightening up and gently stretching from side to side or forward to back. There are a great many opportunities during the day to tip the head and hold it forward. Your awareness in modifying your daily habits to avoid this position will go a long way towards reducing your tendency for head and neck pain.

Because these problems start in youth and are most easily corrected, it is very important to help young people be aware of the potential dangers of poor posture. Rather than just telling them to stand up straight, explain to them how holding their head forward puts a tremendous strain on their neck muscles and vertebrae, creating the stage for painful muscle cramping and possible arthritis.

EXERCISES TO PREVENT PAIN

Regular exercise will help reduce any tendency toward painful muscles spasms of the head and neck. It increases blood flow, thereby reducing the painful build-up of toxins. In addition, exercise strengthens muscles. This gives them a reserve capacity to do work and leaves them less prone to painful spasm from overloading.

When performing the following exercises, a gentle stretching of the muscles is of primary concern. If possible, warm-up the muscles by using moist heat before stretching. However, if heat is not available, don't hesitate to gently perform one or more of these stretching movements occasionally during your daily activities. (Do not forget that without continual restretching, muscles naturally tighten up because of increased stress levels and natural aging. Therefore, once begun, a program of stretching should be continued throughout life.) You should feel a gentle stretch while performing these movements. However, if significant pain develops, you should discontinue these movements and contact your doctor.

Appendix D contains a series of beginning exercises designed to reduce head and neck pain. Once these exercises are mastered without pain, one can consider resuming more strenuous exercise and activity.

THE PREVENTIVE DIET
The area of nutrition, I have found, sometimes can be overwhelming and confusing. When that occurs, the natural tendency is to say: "The heck with it." However, before you give up your desire to develop new eating habits, let me tell you there is good news. There are some simple nutritional guidelines which, when applied over a lifetime, can make a significant difference in the area of head and neck pain.

First and foremost, eliminate caffeine from the diet (coffee, tea, chocolate, regular soft drinks). Second, reduce or eliminate the intake of refined sugars. The tremendous swings in the insulin level caused by the intake of simple sugars and the resulting mood swings between mild hyperactivity and depression can also irritate muscles. In addition, reduce salt consumption. Its effect on the mineral balance of the body and, therefore, of the muscles can cause a tendency toward spasm. Also, moderate or eliminate alcohol consumption. Alcohol's significant effect on the liver, and thus the rest of the body chemistry, also introduces the potential for muscle spasm. Alcohol can also aggravate true migraine headaches, as do a number of food substances. See Appendix C for a listing of these.

It is also important to keep the diet as natural as possible, cooking foods only when necessary. This reduces the intake of artificial products which contain the potential for adverse body reactions and provides higher levels of nutrients through more natural products. Finally, reduce the amount of red meat and increasing the amount of fish in the diet. This reduces the amount of certain compounds which tend to promote inflammation within the body.

ATTITUDE ADJUSTMENT

In the previous chapter on stress, we discussed the importance of being aware of those things within our environment which produce stress. Structural stress, in the area of jaw alignment or head and neck posture, certainly can be a significant cause of head and neck pain. In addition, chemical stressors can also play a significant role in creating the potential for spasm, especially because of their effects on muscle chemistry. Of course, psychological stress also can play an important role in triggering or maintaining head and neck pain.

It is important to remember that our bodies have an amazing ability to adapt to stress. Once that adaptation has occurred, we no longer perceive that we are at a higher stress level. Therefore, as we move up the ladder of greater and greater stress, we often will not be aware of the high tension level we have placed ourselves under. It seems we just "get used to it."

Long-term stress has a potential for eventually breaking down our bodies. Therefore, constant awareness is necessary in order to take steps which reduce our stress levels and keep us healthy.

In addition to the exercises provided in Chapter 7, there are a number of excellent books about stress and stress reduction which can greatly assist you in achieving this goal.

CONCLUSION

There are a number of actions that can be taken in order to prevent head and neck pain and the TM syndrome. Proper maintenance of teeth and elimination of crooked teeth or a bad bite can go a long way towards reducing the structural overload which is often responsible for TM dysfunction-related head and neck pain. In addition, correct head and body posture and care of the muscles which support the head also will help prevent pain. Of course, prudence with regard to ingesting those foods and chemicals which have a profound effect on our body chemistry and the fluid surrounding our muscles, will help keep the muscles healthy and free of painful spasm. Finally, being on guard and aware of the potential for over-stressing ourselves, both physically, chemically and mentally will also reduce the potential for head and neck pain.

The old saying that "an ounce of prevention is worth a pound of cure" can be aptly applied to head and neck pain. A significant percentage of the patients seen for the treatment of head and neck pain probably could have avoided their problem entirely had they known about and followed the recommendations contained in this chapter. Moreover, those patients who have been successfully treated for head and neck pain can more completely insure themselves against its return by following the recommendations presented in this chapter.

One of the most important ways to prevent head and neck pain in adults is to educate children. Because I feel that this is so important, I have devoted one complete chapter to the concept of children and headaches. If we can treat these problems early enough, it is my sincere belief that the epidemic of head and neck pain within his country can be significantly reduced. However, to be successful in this, early recognition and early treatment are absolutely essential. Every parent who suffers this problem should be acutely aware that there is an extremely strong potential that their children will be afflicted by the same pain syndrome. This is due to the fact that many improper structural alignments are hereditary and, therefore, passed on from generation to generation. Thus, it is extremely common for more than one member of a family to suffer from similar head and neck pain problems. However, there is hope. We will discuss this hope in Chapter 11.

CHAPTER 11

Children Can Be Headaches: But They Shouldn't Have Them

Christa was six years old when her mother brought her in for a routine orthodontic examination. Her mother had noticed the crowding of Christa's front teeth. She wanted to know if something could be done at this early age in order to prevent the problem from getting worse. I performed my usual orthodontic examination and also conducted an evaluation for TM dysfunction problems. I did this because my experience has shown me that approximately thirty percent of the children who come to my office for orthodontic treatment have early signs and symptoms of jaw and muscle dysfunction.

As part of my TM dysfunction examination, I asked Christa and her mother if Christa had any headaches. They answered, "Only once or twice a month." I then asked Christa if her jaw got tired when she chewed and she replied "Yes," and added that because of that she did not like to chew gum. Christa's mother was quick to point out that they felt the headaches were sinus headaches, which were fairly common in their family.

As I examined Christa, I noticed a couple of very important clues as to what might be going on with regard to her headaches. First, Christa's face tended to be long and narrow. The distance between her nose and the point of her chin seemed to be a little bit longer than average. This was an extremely strong indication that Christa's lower jaw might be growing more downward than forward, creating a pivot point or fulcrum in the area of the back molars. This was confirmed when I examined Christa's teeth for signs of wear. There was a significant amount of wear on Christa's baby teeth in the back. When I checked for tender muscles, I found that the medial and lateral pterygoid muscle were tender on her left side. This was the same side on which Christa had complained of headaches. Fortunately, there was no noise from the jaw joints themselves, and they were not tender to pressure. I could therefore assume that significant damage had not yet been done to these important structures.

I discussed my suspicion that Christa's headaches might be due to the development of improper jaw alignment as opposed to sinus problems. As I was discussing the progression of this problem which includes, of course, clicking, noisy jaw joints, and frequent head-aches, Christa's mother responded "That's me." She had had head-aches and clicking jaw joints for years. Fortunately, we were able to help both Christa and her mother.

For Christa, we designed an appliance that would relax the jaw muscles and take pressure off of the joint. In addition, the same appliance would begin to redirect the growth of the jaws toward better alignment. For Christa's mother, we fabricated an orthotic splint and proceeded with physical therapy in order to eliminate her headaches, which were much more severe and much more frequent than Christa's.

I t is amazing how frequently I see young patient's with significant early signs of TM problems. Almost as frequently, there is a history in the family of similar problems, usually with one of the parents or even the grandparents. Heredity plays an important role in head and neck pain problems because improper structural alignments, a significant cause of head and neck pain, are passed on from generation to generation. Fortunately, if these problems can be diagnosed and corrected at an early age, long-term results can be freedom from headaches and, very often, a more pleasing facial appearance.

In this chapter, we will see how head and neck pain problems begin to develop in early childhood. In addition, we will examine some of the signs and symptoms which indicate head and neck pain problems are developing. Finally, we will discuss the ways in which this problem can be prevented.

SIGNS OF TROUBLE

In young children, there a number of early signs which indicate that a dysfunction of the jaw structure is beginning to develop. The following is a list of some of these early signs:

Tired jaws	Sore teeth
Headache	Worn teeth
Neck ache	Clicking jaw joints
Earache	Dizziness
Ringing in the ears	Facial deformity

<u>Tired Jaws</u>. Tired jaws are one of the earliest signs that something is wrong with the functioning of the chewing system. The human jaw structure is so well-designed for heavy, repetitive pressure that it is absolutely abnormal for jaws to become tired after chewing. The only reason for this to occur is that the chewing apparatus muscles have become overloaded because of improper jaw alignments. Therefore, any additional work rapidly tires them out. This tiredness will usually occur when eating chewy foods or chewing gum.

I have heard children as young as four years old complain of tired jaws. Upon examination, I have found that significant deviations from normal jaw growth have begun to occur. Of course, many children will not automatically volunteer the information that their jaws are tired. However, when asked, they will relay this information, often giving specific examples. Should tiredness of the jaw occur, the child should immediately be evaluated by a professional trained in the area of TM dysfunction.

Headaches. Headaches are a significant sign that a TM problem is beginning to develop. It is important to remember that headache pain is not normal, especially in young children. Normally, they are healthy and have relatively low stress levels. Therefore, headaches that do occur are usually a sign that their system is significantly overloaded. The headaches do not have to be frequent to be a sign of problems. Headaches as little as once or twice a month can be an early warning sign and, therefore, should be taken seriously. Of course, there are other things beside TM dysfunction, such as visual disturbances, that can create headaches in children. However, when the cause is not easily correctable or obvious, a TM dysfunction problem should be suspected.

Neck aches. Neck aches can also be a significant sign that TM dysfunction problems are developing. Poor posture alone, or combined with a developing TM problem, can significantly over-load neck muscles creating pain and discomfort. With many of our children, posture tends to deteriorate as they mature. Thus, neck aches become more frequent in susceptible individuals as children move into their teenage years. Early evaluation, diagnosis, education, and treatment for these problems can go a long way toward providing a lifetime of better health and comfort for these young individuals.

Earaches. Earaches are not uncommon in young children. Often they are the result of chronic ear infection or blockage of the eustachian tube, which allows air pressure to equalize between the external environment and the middle ear. There a number of ways in which earaches can be related to dysfunctions of the jaws. Very often, pain will be referred to the ear area, when, in fact, the irritated area is not the ear but the jaw joint or one or more of the surrounding muscles. This referred pain is a very common source of earache, both in children and adults. In addition, the opening of the eustachian tube, which drains the middle ear is in an area surrounded by a muscle. When this muscle is in spasm, it affects the eustachian tube and pressure and fluid can begin to build-up in the middle ear. This muscle can go into spasm any time there is spasm in the jaw muscles, because all of these structures develop from the same early tissues in the embryo, and, consequently, their nerves are closely related. Needless to say, an earache should be evaluated by the family physician. However, if earaches become frequent or occur in combination with any of the other signs which we are discussing in this section, examination a professional trained in the area of TM dysfunction problems should be sought.

Ringing in the Ears. Tinnitus, the medical term for ringing in the ears, can have a number of causes and should always be evaluated by a physician. However, if a medical cause cannot be determined, there is a strong possibility that it is being caused by a spasm in the tensor tympanic muscle of the middle ear. This will also cause fluctuations in the hearing level. As with the muscle around the eustachian tube, this muscle can also go into spasm when the chewing muscles are irritated because the two come from the same embryological area. Approximately fifty percent of the adult patients who come into to my office and have ringing in the ears, leave with no ringing in the ears after treatment for TM problems. If children report that their ears are ringing, they should first be evaluated by a physician. However, if a cause is not found or if significant other signs of TM dysfunction problems exist, they also should have a TM evaluation.

Sore Teeth. Sore teeth are another sign that something is not right with the chewing mechanism. It is not normal for teeth to be sore unless the tooth is undergoing some degenerative change or is being overloaded due to a severe clenching habit or an improper structural alignment. Even children who tend to clench their teeth will not normally have sore teeth, unless tooth alignment is off enough to create significant overload in one specific area. If children complain of sore teeth, they should be evaluated immediately by their dentist so that the cause can be determined!

Worn Teeth. Worn teeth are an extremely significant sign that there is an incorrect alignment of the jaw structure. Years ago, dentists assumed that the baby teeth in some individuals just wore out because they were weak or because the patient tended to clench and grind a lot. Recent research indicates that this may not be the case. When teeth or jaws are improperly aligned, the body unconsciously wants to remove the offending tooth parts. Thus, a pattern of grinding and clenching may be initiated. Unfortunately, because of the position of some teeth and the neurological dominance of others, the offending portion may not necessarily be the area that wears down.

Very often, the first person to notice this wearing down of teeth will be the family dentist. However, parents can examine their children's teeth. Normal teeth will have very sharp points on the back teeth or a slight unevenness or bumps on the edges of the front teeth. If these points or bumps are worn off, this is a sign of trouble! There should be very little or no sign of significantly flattened or polished areas on the teeth. Should either of these problems occur, an improper structural alignment is very likely at fault and the early seeds of a TM dysfunction problem are being sown.

Clicking Jaw Joints. Noisy jaw joints are a cardinal sign that jaw dysfunction is developing. No matter how infrequently the click occurs, this problem should be immediately evaluated by a professional trained in the area of TM problems. I have seen five-year-old children with clicking jaws. That means that there already has been significant stretching and damage to the ligaments of the joint. Fortunately, if this problem is treated at an early age, there is an excellent likelihood that the joints will tighten up because of the

physical resiliency of healthy, young, growing individuals. However, if these problems are not treated early, the probability of a
completely slipped disc, and eventual arthritic degeneration in the
joints at a fairly early age, is very likely.

Dizziness. This can also be a sign that a structural imbalance is
developing. Since there are serious problems that could be related
to dizziness, it is best that a physician evaluate the problem at first.
However, should the dizziness persist, or should it be combined
with any of the other signs we have listed thus far, an evaluation
for TM dysfunction should be undertaken. Very often, dizziness
associated with jaw dysfunction occurs because of spasm in the
neck muscles which contain balance receptors. Irritation in these
muscles causes a signal to be sent to the brain which does not match
those received through the eyes and dizziness, not unlike that
which is experienced when a person is seasick, occurs.

As we have seen in previous chapters, any malfunction and
overload in the jaw muscles often will tend to aggravate the neck
muscles. This is why TM dysfunction problems should always be
evaluated when persistent dizziness occurs. (It would be interesting
to study those people who are prone to seasickness to see if they
also tend to have inflammation or trigger areas within the neck
musculature.)

Facial Deformity. I have included facial deformity in this section,
because, frequently, a person who has an unfavorable facial growth
pattern will eventually develop dysfunction of the jaw joint and
head and neck muscles. When the muscles are finally overloaded
enough, it becomes only a matter of time before symptoms appear.
Therefore, if a child's lower jaw is protruding forward, if the upper
jaw is ahead of the lower, or if the face seems to be growing off to
one side or the other, immediate attention and evaluation is
required by an orthodontist who is trained to deal with correction
of facial growth problems. Failure to do so at an early age may

condemn the child to future jaw surgery in order to correct the problem.

In the next section, I would like to deal with some easy concepts regarding facial growth and how significant it is with regard to head and neck pain problems.

GROWING FOR BETTER OR FOR WORSE

I cannot overemphasize how important the growth pattern of the upper and lower jaw is in relationship to the development of head and neck pain. After years of treating this type of problem, very often I can look at a person and tell if they are going to have clicking jaw joints and headache problems. Unfortunately, both the medical and dental professions are just beginning to understand how important jaw alignment is to the total well-being of the head and neck muscles. Until this information is more widely understood and distributed, a great deal of head and neck pain will be misunderstood and improperly diagnosed.

As a child grows, a relationship is established between the position of the upper and lower jaw, both in a front to back and in an up and down direction. For example, if there is insufficient growth of the lower jaw in a horizontal direction, it will appear as if the upper teeth stick out and the lower teeth are back. In order for the child to maintain normal swallowing and speech patterns, the lower jaw will need to be brought forward much more than is normal. This causes a number of facial muscles required to pull the jaw forward to become overloaded. Combine this with muscles which become irritated in order to protect teeth which bump, and the net effect is the development of chronic muscle spasm and headache.

To make matters worse, a pivot point may develop in the back of the mouth which is destructive to the temporomandibular joint. (See Chapter 5, Figure 5.2) Unfortunately, in many instances it takes years of chronic overload for actual pain problems to develop. At that point, a great deal of growth may have been completed. It is, therefore, extremely important to recognize the early signs and symptoms of this problem so that appropriate measures may be undertaken to redirect the growth of the jaws. However, once the jaw bones have been completely formed, it often becomes necessary to reposition them by means of surgery.

GROWTH OF THE JAW JOINT

In addition to abnormalities in the positioning of the two jaws, the jaw joint itself may begin to develop an undesirable shape. This occurs because the joint will grow improperly in order to adapt to poor tooth and jaw positions. The temporomandibular joint does not reach its complete adult size and shape until the child is approximately seven years of age. Before this time, it is under the influence of the developing jaw and tooth positions. Thus, if the front teeth overlap, creating what is termed a deep bite, the sides of the jaw joint will accommodate this improper tooth position by becoming very steep. This creates a problem mechanically for the joint because, when the walls of the joint are very steep, the condyle, or lower jaw, does not travel easily in and out of its socket. This causes excessive mechanical pressures within the joint. Thus, it is not uncommon for individuals with a deep bite to have clicking and pain develop in the jaw joints. If this overlapping of the front teeth can be avoided or eliminated during the time that the joint is reaching its final shape (approximately five to seven years of age), the joint will not assume this deep, steep-sided contour and mechanical pressure within the joint can be reduced. Consequently, the possibility of headache pain due to jaw dysfunction in later life is reduced.

On the other hand, in those children who have a long, narrow face where the lower jaw is growing vertically, an open bite will often be evident between the front teeth. Because of the posterior fulcrum or pivot which is created (See Chapter 5, Figure 5.2), the condyle of the lower jaw does not develop sufficiently. This often results in a weak joint. Insufficient development of the condyle is most often due to a lack of sufficient pressure in the proper direction which would stimulate sufficient bone growth and shape.

Our knowledge regarding the influence of tooth position and jaw structure upon the development of the jaw joints is just beginning to unfold. As we learn more about the relationship between the two, even more effective methods of treatment can be developed. At present, the best policy seems to be correction of these problems as early as possible in order to minimize a the long-term impact of poor jaw structure upon the developing joint.

POSTURE: STAND UP STRAIGHT

"Stand up straight" is one of the things my father used to tell me when I was a youngster. Although he was unable to explain the medical reason for doing so, he and a great many others in his generation knew that standing up straight would lessen the chances for back pain.

Of course, by now the reader already has significant knowledge about the relationship of poor posture to strain of head and neck muscles. It is important to remember that these problems start at a very early age. As time goes on, muscles and ligaments take a more permanent shape which makes correction more difficult. Over time, these chronically improperly positioned structures can tend to create arthritic changes in the vertebrae of the neck. Therefore, early correction—proper posture along with exercises as necessary—can help reduce the tendency for head and neck pain throughout an individual's life.

NUTRITIONAL CONSIDERATIONS

Unfortunately, the diet of today's youth is often appallingly incomplete. Fast foods and junk foods are notoriously high in fat and low in essential nutrients. Moreover, the heavy consumption of sweets creates the potential for muscle spasm and also significantly reduces the body's store of vitamin C, which is essential for maintaining the strength and adequate growth of ligaments and tissues. When we consider the potential impact of adequate nutrition upon the regeneration and growth of the cartilage within the joint structure, it is frightening to think that the seeds of arthritic degeneration may be sown at such an early age.

One of the significant findings that surgeons see when exploring malfunctioning jaw joints in adults and young patients as well as a stickiness or a loss of lubrication within the joint structure. There is a strong possibility that this stickiness is due to overloading of the joints along with other chemical factors, one of which may be a lack of sufficient vitamin C within the surrounding tissue. Without sufficient tissue levels of vitamin C, overloading within the joints from structural problems activates the enzyme called hyaluronidase which destroys joint lubrication. With high vitamin C tissue levels this enzyme is inhibited and the joint retains its lubrication. Moreover, a poor diet may increase the potential damage from waste products in the joint due to a lack of anti-oxidant vitamins in the tissue. This, again, points to the probability that the seeds of later arthritic degeneration are being sown at an early age.

Children, in general, but especially those children who are prone to head and neck pain problems—or who have parents that have suffered from head and neck pain problems—should be taught about the relationship of diet and nutrition to pain. Children should be instructed to eat a good breakfast, since not doing so will cause a drop in blood sugar at approximately mid-morning, creating a headache. They should also be taught about the significant, harmful effects of a high-sugar diet upon the body as a whole and, in particular, the muscle structure and ligaments. Children also should be taught the advantages of taking a multiple vitamin supplement in order to insure proper nutritional coverage. Finally, they should be made aware of the advantages of consuming more fish in their diet as opposed to red meat, thereby reducing the amount of animal fat in the diet.

As a parent working with his own family, the author has found that gentle instruction rather than preaching and living the lifestyle which you would like your child to emulate are the most effective ways to have children develop good habits. In addition, a warm, supporting relationship with a professional who is trained in the area of dealing with head and neck pain problems will go a long way toward encouraging youngsters to improve their health habits.

CONCLUSION

It is a tragedy that so many young people endure significant amounts of head and neck pain when the prevention and cure of these problems is much easier at an early age. When one considers that headache pain is the primary, most significant cause of workdays lost in the United States, the cost to human productivity that could be saved through the early detection and correction of these problems is considerable indeed. Through the simple use of orthotics, combined with various appliances by which orthodontists are able to influence the magnitude and direction of jaw growth, much suffering and discomfort could be eliminated.

One major difficulty facing parents of children who have these problems developing is that many physicians and dentists practicing today were not trained in the diagnosis and treatment of these problems. Therefore, it is important for the parent to seek out those practitioners who have had significant post-graduate training in these areas. With the help of such skilled individuals, head and neck pain can be eliminated or greatly reduced without the use of drugs or surgery.

In the final chapter of this book, I would like to share with you some frequently asked questions and their answers, some of which I hope you will find pertinent to your own situation or the situation of another who is close to you.

CHAPTER 12

Questions and Answers

Q. I have been told that I have arthritis in my neck. Is there any relationship between my neck pain and a possible jaw alignment problem?

A. If x-rays were taken which demonstrate degeneration of the bones of the neck, you most certainly have arthritis. However, many people can have significant degeneration of the bones in the neck with little or no pain, since most neck pain arises from muscle spasm and trigger points within the muscles. This being the case, therapy directed at improving posture and work habits and at eliminating trigger points through physical therapy and stretching can go a long way toward significantly reducing or eliminating neck pain.

Unfortunately, in some instances, x-rays have not been taken. Patients have been told that their pain is likely due to arthritis in the neck. The problem, however, may be merely due to muscle spasm and tightness. When neck pain is treated, its relationship to dysfunction in the chewing apparatus is often overlooked. Since a dynamic balance exists between the muscles of our body, overload in any one particular area will cause a change in the tension of associated and opposing muscles. If the facial muscles become more tense due to problems in the bite arise from improperly aligned teeth or jaws, the neck muscles increase their tension in order to compensate for the tension in the front of the head. If this were not so, our head would gradually begin to tip farther and farther forward. As you can imagine, this increase in tension of the neck muscles will aggravate any overloading of the muscles already present, triggering neck pain. In addition, pain may be referred to the neck from an inflamed jaw joint or chewing muscle.

Q. What is a migraine personality and how is it related to head and neck pain?

A. The term *migraine personality* has been used to described those people who tend to create higher stress levels in their lives through being ambitious and perfectionistic. The temptation, when this type of label is applied, is to ignore the underlying structural factors that may be overloading the muscles of the head and neck and, instead, concentrating only on the psychological aspects involved. For that reason, it is extremely important that patients be aware not only of their tendency toward creating internal stress but also to the fact that underlying structural causes may be at the root of the problem.

Q. Why doesn't aspirin get rid of my headaches?

A. Aspirin and most over-the-counter painkillers can provide a great deal of relief for minor pain problems. However, the head and neck pain that many people are subject to is of a more severe nature. As a matter of fact, in my own experience I have seen patients who required heavy doses of narcotics to a severe episode of jaw joint or muscle spasm pain.

Q. I have been diagnosed as having migraines. How can I tell if there is a relationship between my headache pain and my jaw structure?

A. Many patients who have been diagnosed as migraine sufferers have problems related directly to the malfunction of their chewing apparatus. These problems are often difficult to diagnose and, frequently, require the actual placement of an orthotic splint to determine if help can be provided. For this reason, I usually consider the first month or two of orthotic splint therapy as a diagnostic period. During this time, we can determine the patient's response to possible treatment measures. My experience has been that over fifty percent of the patients who arrive in my office with a diagnosis of migraine headaches, in fact, have never had a migraine at all. Because of the difficulty in accurately diagnosing these types of problems, I feel that it would be wise for any chronic migraine sufferer to have an evaluation by a professional well-trained in the diagnosis and treatment of TM dysfunction.

Q. I have sinus problems and so does my family. This couldn't be related to my jaw, or could it?

A. There is a muscle located deep within the mouth called the external pterygoid muscle. When this muscle becomes inflamed, pain will often be felt (referred) under the eyes in the area of the sinus. Unfortunately, an extremely high percentage of so called sinus headache is actually due to the pain generated by this inflamed muscle, which became inflamed due to ill-fitting teeth and/or a clenching habit.

same type of headache that I do. It seems
ion headache. Can these be hereditary?

on headaches are often related to improp-
eeth, there is a strong tendency for them
...ary. This is true because we inherit the shape of our
jaws, and even the position of our teeth, from our parents. For
example, if your mother has a long narrow face and you also
have a long narrow face, the chances of your having a fulcrum
or pivot on the back molars, thus creating pain, is very likely.

Q. I've heard that TM dysfunction problems require surgery. I've
also heard that surgery should be avoided. What is accurate?

A. A very small percentage of patients having TM dysfunction
requires surgery on the jaw joint. However, since this problem
is often caused by an improperly aligned jaw structure, the need
for surgery to realign the jaws is more likely, although the
number of patients requiring this kind of surgery is still rather
low. Fortunately, most patients can be maintained in a comfortable state without surgery on the joint or surgery to reposition
the jaws.

Q. Do injured jaw joints ever heal?

A. In youngsters and teenagers the probability that injuries to the
jaw joints will heal is very good. However, as we age the healing
process within the joints becomes diminished. Moreover,
stretched ligaments heal very slowly, and often not at all. This
results in chronic clicks within the joint. Because of this, many
patients who have damaged joints, due to accidents or trauma
from a poor bite, will never have joints "like new" again.
However, with proper management these patients can lead a
normal relatively pain-free existence.

Q. I've been told that headache pain is all in my head?

A. Of course, it is true that head pain is in fact "in your head." Unfortunately, what is really meant by this statement is that the pain is not real; it is psychogenic. This diagnosis is often made when a better more appropriate one cannot be found. It is sad; but many patients have been condemned to a life of pain and constant medication because of this label. My experience shows that for the majority of patients there is a structural or organic cause for their pain.

Q. Can foods cause headaches?

A. There are a number of foods that have been implicated in causing migraines: wines, aged cheeses, chocolates, salt, and excessive alcohol intake are some. (See Appendix C) In addition, the food additive MSG (monosodium glutamate) has been known to cause headache pain, creating the so called "Chinese food" headache. (Chinese food contains MSG). In addition, hard, crunchy, or chewy foods can also aggravate an already inflamed muscle structure or temporomandibular joint. Therefore, whenever I suspect TM dysfunction I always recommend a soft diet for the first week or two of treatment.

Q. I've noticed a difficulty in speaking, since I developed what my dentist calls TM dysfunction headaches. Is this possible, and if so how?

A. Speaking is a extremely sophisticated muscular movement. Thus, whenever there are spasms in the chewing muscles there also is a possibility that speaking will be impaired, especially if the muscles underneath the lower jaw are tense. In addition, remember that the tongue itself is muscle. Therefore, it can be affected by spasms in the surrounding musculature. It is not unusual to have changes in one's speaking ability, especially if severe headache pain is involved. Fortunately, when the muscle spasms are brought under control, speaking returns to normal rather rapidly.

Q. Is it possible to have changes in vision with TM dysfunction headaches?

A. Although we do not understand the exact mechanism, a number of studies have shown slight changes in the iris of the eye when sufficient facial muscle spasm is present. In addition, due to what is called *autonomic response*, the eyes may also weep when the surrounding muscle structural is irritated. Incidentally, the nose may run under these circumstances. A runny nose and weeping eyes mimic an allergic reaction, sometimes making diagnosis more difficult.

Q. I recently had an orthotic made to help my headaches, and not only did my headaches get better but my lower back pain was also sufficiently reduced. Are these two related?

A. There is a system of muscles from our hips all the way up to the back of the head. Each muscle preforms a specific task and relies on other muscles around it to aid it in its function. When any one of these muscles becomes inflamed and irritated, it will affect the dynamic balance of the others. It is probably not likely that a TM dysfunction headache could cause a lower back problem. However, in a situation where there is already overloading and compromise in the lower back area, even a slight change of position in the head due to a muscle spasm could trigger lower back pain.

CONCLUSION

We have explored the relationship of head and neck pain to dysfunction and improper alignment of the jaws and their supporting structures. From birth through adulthood any event, be it growth and development or trauma, which results in improperly aligned jaws or teeth can eventually create muscle spasm. Muscle spasm is Mother Nature's way of reducing the movement of the injured parts in order to prevent further injury.

We have seen how the abuse of the jaw structure can be unlimited, due to the fact that it has the only set of joints in the human body which never requires rest. We have also seen how nutrition can have an effect, either positively or negatively, upon the healing of these structures. We have examined the "Great Impostor," TM dysfunction, which effects as many as one-out-of-four Americans.

The good news is that we are making progress in the diagnosis and treatment of TM dysfunction problems. Unfortunately, misunderstanding or lack of knowledge keeps many people from obtaining help. This book has been written in the hope that it will provide help for the many who have suffered with head and neck pain and also will provide help for those who now may be growing into headaches.

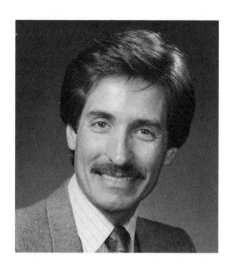

ABOUT THE AUTHOR

D r. Randall Moles received his Doctor of Dental Science (D.D.S.) degree with honors in 1970 and his Master's Degree in orthodontics in 1974 from Marquette University. He has served on the faculty of Marquette University as Associate Clinical Professor of Orthodontics and is frequently asked to return as a guest lecturer.

Dr. Moles is actively engaged in the fields of orthodontics and the treatment of head and neck pain. Over the years, he has brought relief from pain and better dental health to hundreds of individuals, in addition to teaching these techniques to his colleagues in dentistry. He is also involved in research and development of new products for the orthodontics field. One such product is a custom designed scuba mouthpiece to eliminate jaw discomfort and headache pain for divers.

Dr. Moles practices in Racine, Wisconsin, located on the shore of Lake Michigan near Chicago and Milwaukee. (Professionals interested in courses or consultations with Dr. Moles can reach him at 5801 Washington Ave., Racine, WI 53406, (414)884-7700).

APPENDIX A

Self-examination for Head and Neck Pain

The following procedures, when performed on you by you, *may* indicate to you whether or not you have any of the common TM dysfunction symptoms.

1. PRESS ON THE TM JOINT. Pressure applied to the TM joint should not be painful. If pain is present, inflammation may be present and headaches may result.

2. CHECK FOR CLICKS AND GRINDS. Open wide and close your mouth a number of times. Then move your jaw as far as it will move from side-to-side. The movements should be smooth and no noise should result. If clicking or grinding is heard, that is a indication that a TM dysfunction problem is present.

3. CHECK THE MOUTH OPENING. Use the *three finger test* to check for an adequate jaw opening. You should be able to get three of the knuckles on your non-dominant hand between your upper and lower front teeth when your mouth is open. If you are

unable to do this, that is an indication that a TM dysfunction problem may be present.

4. CHECK THE OPENING AND CLOSING PATTERN. Look at yourself in the mirror while opening and closing your mouth. Notice whether or not your lower jaw is moving straight up and down. If it deviates or wiggles from side-to-side, that is an indication that a TM dysfunction problem may be present.

5. CHECK OVERLAP OF FRONT TEETH. If the front teeth do not touch, or if the upper teeth greatly overlap the lower teeth, a TM dysfunction problem may be present.

7. CHECK TOOTH ALIGNMENT. Crooked teeth can cause protective responses in the muscles which lead to TM dysfunction problems.

8. CHECK FOR WORN TEETH. Look closely at your upper and lower teeth, both in the front and in the back of your mouth. If any noticeable wear is present, a TM dysfunction problem may be present.

> NOTE: The more recent and severe a headache is, the more dangerous it is and the greater the possibility that a severe medical problem could exist. Under such circumstances, contact your physician immediately.

APPENDIX B

What to Do When
Chronic Headaches Strike

1. LIMIT JAW OPENING AND MOVEMENT. If muscles or joints are inflamed, using them will only make matters worse. Therefore, chew, talk, and use your mouth as little as possible.

2. BEGIN A SOFT DIET. If muscles and joints are irritated a softer diet will reduce the strain on already aggravated structures.

3. MOIST HEAT. The application of moist heat, using warm towels or a moist heating pad, can help reduce muscle spasm and inflammation. When applying heat, make sure to wrap the heating pad or the moist towel around the back of the neck up and forward toward the jaw area. In this way, many potentially irritated muscles can be covered.

4. REST. If possible, lie down and rest. This relaxation will help reduce muscle spasm.

REMEMBER: These measures may help to reduce or eliminate headache pain. However, it is important to have a thorough evaluation so that underlying structural problems can be corrected. Failure to do so could lead to more significant problems later, such as increasingly severe headaches, loss of teeth, and arthritis in the temporomandibular joints.

APPENDIX C

Foods and Drinks That May Cause Headaches

Milk and Cheese
Chocolate
Herring
Fermented foods (pickled
  or marinated)
Sour cream
Yogurt
Vinegar
Freshly baked products
Nuts
Monosodium glutamate
  (MSG)
Peas
Raw beans

Onions
Canned figs
Bananas
Citrus fruits
Pork
Carbonated beverages
Avocados
Fermented sausage
Cured meats
Chicken livers
Wine
Alcohol
Beer

APPENDIX D

The following exercises should be performed slowly and rhythmically. NOTE: It is best to warm the muscles with moist heat for fifteen to twenty minutes prior to preforming these exercises. A warm stretching feeling may be felt during the exercises. If pain develops, the exercise should be discontinued, and a professional should be contacted for guidance.

These exercises should be faithfully performed on a daily basis, and each exercise should be repeated six times.

EXERCISE 1
UNDER SHOWER STRETCH

This exercise is used to stretch the muscles in the back of the head. Ideally, it should be done while sitting on a small stool in a warm shower. However, it can be done without the stool.

While sitting on the stool in a warm shower (see Figure 1), bring the hands behind the head, clasping the fingers. Gently pull the head forward and downward while relaxing the neck muscles. The weight of the head and the hands will gently provide stretch. You then can move the head slowly, side to side, in rotation movements to stretch all the muscle bands.

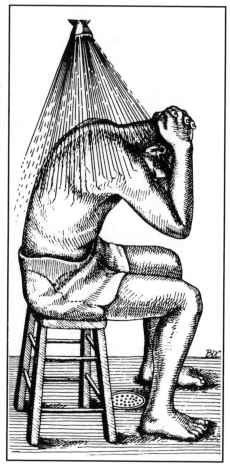

Figure 1

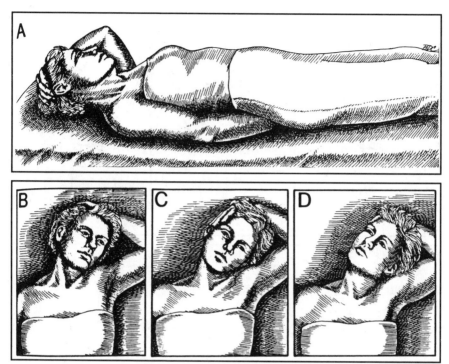

Figure 2

EXERCISE 2
SIDE BENDING NECK EXERCISE

This exercise should be performed while lying down. One hand is anchored under the buttock, while the other hand is placed on top of the head. Gently pull the head away from the side to be stretched. (In Figure 2-B, the face is turned toward the direction of pull.) Then move the head upright. In Figure 2-C, the patient looks forward during the stretching movement, after which the head is brought upright. And in Figure 2-D, the face is turned away from the direction of pull, after which the head is brought upright. By moving into three different positions, three different muscle groups are stretched. The same procedure should be applied to the opposite side, reversing hands and positions.

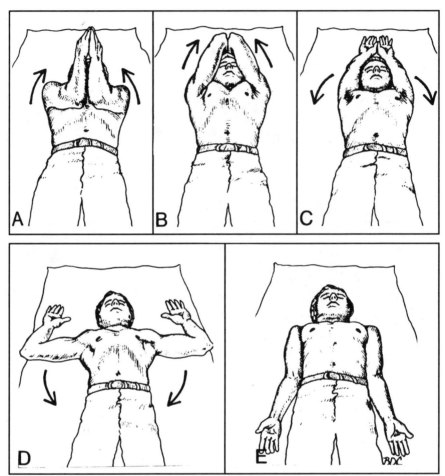

Figure 3

EXERCISE 3
UPPER BACK STRETCH

This exercise should be performed while lying down in a relaxed position. Bring the arms together as in Figure 3-A. Rotate the arms up over the head as in Figure 3-B. Straighten the arms above the head as in Figure 3-C. Bring the arms down while bending at the elbow, as in Figure 3-D, and straighten the arms out and relax as in Figure 3-E. Upon completion, rest for 15 seconds while breathing deeply.

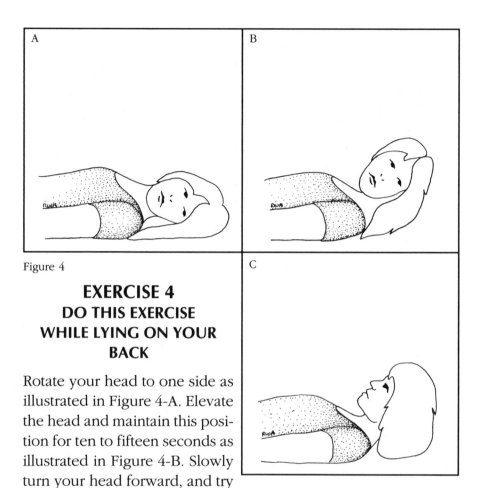

Figure 4

EXERCISE 4
DO THIS EXERCISE WHILE LYING ON YOUR BACK

Rotate your head to one side as illustrated in Figure 4-A. Elevate the head and maintain this position for ten to fifteen seconds as illustrated in Figure 4-B. Slowly turn your head forward, and try to touch your chin to your chest as shown in illustration Figure 4-C. Slowly lower your head down and relax for thirty seconds. Repeat this exercise in the opposite direction.

EXERCISE 5
NECK ROTATION

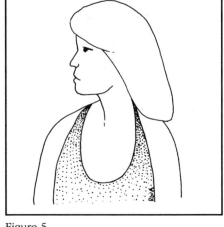

This exercise should be done while standing or sitting in a relaxed body posture. (See Figure 5) Keeping the head level, gently rotate your head to the right as far as possible without causing pain. Maintain this position for fifteen seconds. (Note: It is important to maintain a level head position). Relax for fifteen

Figure 5

seconds. Then rotate your head to the left as far as possible without causing pain.

EXERCISE 6
SIDE BENDING

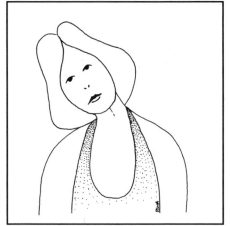

This exercise is very similar to EXERCISE 1 and can be performed either sitting or standing in a relaxed position. As in Figure 6, slowly bend your head to

Figure 6

one side and try to touch your shoulder with your ear. (NOTE: It is important not to raise your shoulder during this procedure). Maintain this position for fifteen seconds. Then relax for fifteen seconds. This exercise then should be repeated in the opposite direction.

EXERCISE 7
NECK RAISING EXTENSION

This exercise can be performed in a relaxed sitting or standing position. As in Figure 7, raise your head and point your chin toward the ceiling; hold this position for fifteen to twenty seconds. Bring your head forward into a neutral position and relax for fifteen seconds.

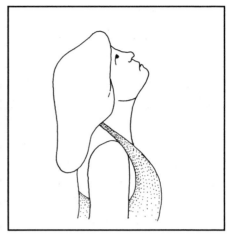

Figure 7

EXERCISE 8
NECK LOWERING

With your teeth together, lower your chin so that it touches your chest. (See Figure 8) Maintain this position for fifteen seconds, slowly raise your head to a neutral position, and then relax for fifteen seconds.

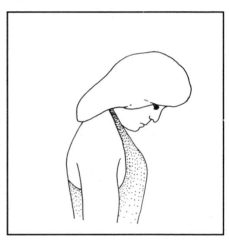

Figure 8

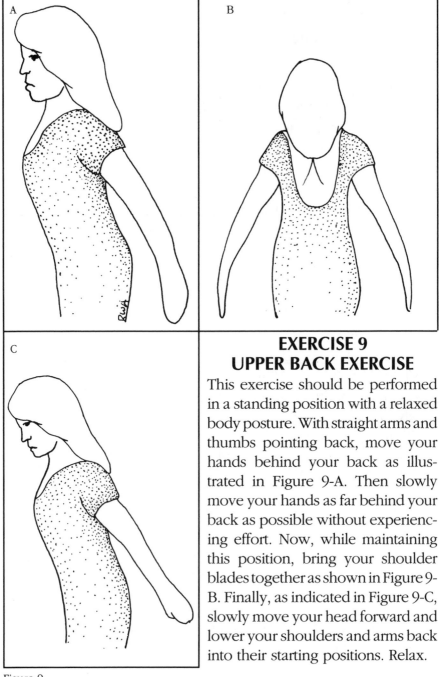

EXERCISE 9
UPPER BACK EXERCISE

This exercise should be performed in a standing position with a relaxed body posture. With straight arms and thumbs pointing back, move your hands behind your back as illustrated in Figure 9-A. Then slowly move your hands as far behind your back as possible without experiencing effort. Now, while maintaining this position, bring your shoulder blades together as shown in Figure 9-B. Finally, as indicated in Figure 9-C, slowly move your head forward and lower your shoulders and arms back into their starting positions. Relax.

Figure 9

BIBLIOGRAPHY

Benson, Herbert, M.D. *The Relaxation Response.* New York: William Morrow and Company, 1975.

Dufty, William. *Sugar Blues.* New York: Warner Books, 1975.

Hanson, Peter G., M.D. *The Joy of Stress.* New York: Andrews, McMeel & Parker, 1986.

Jafe, Dennis T. Ph.D. *Healing From Within.* New York: Simon & Schuster, 1980.

Padus, Emrika. *The Complete Guide to Your Emotions & Your Health.* Emmaus: Rodale Press, 1986.

Pelletier, Kenneth R. *Mind as Healer Mind as Slayer.* New York: Del Publishing Co., 1977.

Selye, Hans M.D. *Stress Without Distress.* New York: Harper & Row, 1974.

Travell, Janet G., M.D. and David G. Simons. *Myofascial Pain and Dysfunction: The Trigger Point Manual.* Maryland: Williams and Wilkins, 1983.

Wright, Jonathan V., M.D. *Dr. Wright's Guide to Healing with Nutrition.* Emmaus: Rodale Press, 1984.

INDEX

Here's What People Are Saying After Reading
ENDING HEAD AND NECK PAIN:

"Wonderful! As one who has suffered from this problem for many years, I found it immensely useful!"

Janice S. Gruninger
Registered Dietitian
St. Mary's/Mayo Clinic

"In the present day, when the general public deserves and demands more information concerning their own health problems, this book comes highly recommended. It is also encouraged reading for the medical practitioner, whose knowledge always needs updating."

E. W. Waldeck, M.D.
Assistant Clinical Professor
Ophthamology
Medical College of Wisconsin

"This timely publication offers the public a broad overview of a vast and complicated subject; it is highly recommended for patients and dentists alike who are involved with temporomandibular joint disorders!"

Donald E. Romsa, D.D.S.
Assistant Clinical Professor
Oral and Maxillofacial Surgery
Northwestern University Medical
Center/Chicago

"Dr. Moles has made an important contribution to both practitioners and patients by creating a comprehensive new framework in which to view the problem of recurrent headaches."

Thomas L. Beck
President and CEO
Unico, Inc.

IF YOU HAVE FREQUENT HEAD AND NECK PAIN, YOU NEED TO KNOW:
* How improperly aligned teeth and jaws can create muscle spasm and headaches . . .
* How severe headache pain can be relieved without drugs . . .
* How muscles become chronically irritated and how stress triggers pain . . .

Order Coupon

MOLES PUBLISHING DIVISION
5801 Washington Ave., Ste. 100
Racine, WI 53406
Fax 414-884-7710   THANK YOU!
Office 414-884-7700

Please send me _____ copies of ENDING HEAD AND NECK PAIN: THE TMJ CONNECTION.

NAME _____

ADDRESS _____

CITY _____

STATE _____

_____ books / $12.95 = $_____

**Shipping = _____

(Wisconsin residents only) Sales Tax = _____

(Add $.65 per item)

TOTAL = _____

**Shipping

( ) UPS - Allow 6-7 working days for delivery.
Include: $4.25 for 1st item
$1.25 for each additional

( ) USPS Special 4th Class - Allow 10-14 working days for delivery.
Include: $3.25 per item.

ENCLOSED IS MY CHECK FOR: $_____

Here is my VISA/MASTER CARD number. Please charge my account.

VISA_____

Master Card_____

Expiration Date_____

Signature_____